'*The Tyranny of Health* should be kept by the bed as an indispensable second opinion and an antidote to health panics past, present and future.'

Mick Hume, *The New Statesman*

'This is a powerful book.... It is as much a crisp analysis of the decline of libertarian values among the political left as it is a damning critique of health provision in Britain.... *The Tyranny of Health* expresses with great clarity and precision the growing sense of unease that many people, both inside and outside the medical profession, are beginning to experience.'

Social Issues Research Centre, Oxford

'This is a wide-ranging book which draws together many of the key issues in contemporary health policy and general medical practice, placing them in the context of broader social and political changes ... a very persuasive and enjoyable text.'

Dr David Wainwright, *International Epidemiology*

'Fitzpatrick's conclusion is unnerving: the recommendations for changes in lifestyle, the increasingly intrusive screening procedures, and the impertinent offers of advice on domestic violence, sexual abuse, defective parenting and so forth, add up to doctors no longer practising medicine. Instead, the medical profession is "at the cutting edge of the drive to extend professional regulation over personal life". It is important that we question these developments and this book offers an excellent starting point.'

Stuart W.G. Derbyshire, University of Pittsburgh Medical Centre, *British Medical Journal*

'There is no area of life that could not be subsumed under the headings Health or PsychoSocial if the State found that convenient. *The Tyranny of Health* is a most important and timely book and everyone concerned with health and care should read it.'

Derek Steinberg, psychiatrist, *Holistic Health*

THE TYRANNY OF HEALTH

Doctors and the regulation of lifestyle

Michael Fitzpatrick

London and New York

First published 2001
by Routledge
11 New Fetter Lane, London EC4P 4EE

Simultaneously published in the USA and Canada
by Routledge
29 West 35th Street, New York, NY 10001

Reprinted 2001

Routledge is an imprint of the Taylor & Francis Group

Typeset in Times by Taylor & Francis Books Ltd
Printed and bound in Great Britain by Biddles Ltd,
Guildford and King's Lynn

British Library Cataloguing in Publication Data
A catalogue record for this book is available from the British Library

Library of Congress Cataloging in Publication Data
Fitzpatrick, Michael, 1950–
The tyranny of health: doctors and the regulation of lifestyle /
Michael Fitzpatrick.
Includes bibliographical references and index.
1. Medicine–Political aspects–Great Britain. 2. Medical policy–Great
Britain. 3. Medical care–political aspects–Great Britain. I. Title.
RA395.G6 F586 2000
362.1''0941 21; aa05 06–05–dc00
00-042470

ISBN 0–415–23571–5 (hbk)
ISBN 0–415–23572–3 (pbk)

CONTENTS

PREFACE

On a bitterly cold February day in the winter of 1987 I had to break into the house of an elderly couple who had succumbed to a combination of infection and hypothermia. While I waited for the ambulance I found, unopened on the doormat, a copy of the government's 'Don't Die of Ignorance' leaflet which had been distributed to twenty-three million households as part of the campaign to alert the nation to the danger of Aids. Around half of these households contained either an old couple or an old person living alone. (One elderly woman in Dorset wrote to a national newspaper inquiring 'do you think this caring government would swap my Aids leaflet (as new) for a bucket of coal?' *Guardian* 15 January 1987.) While this experience brought home the absurdity of the 'everyone is at risk' campaign, several encounters in my surgery in the same period with people in a state of fear about Aids who were at low (if not zero) risk of HIV infection, made me wonder whether there was something more insidious about the whole campaign.

What was striking about the 'worried well' was not only the intensity of their anxiety about a rare disease that they had little chance of contracting, but the effect of the Aids publicity in making them question the way they conducted their personal life. Whether or not they were at risk of HIV, the Aids campaign put people under real pressure to conform to official guidelines regarding their most intimate relationships. The more I examined the Aids campaign the less it seemed to be a rational response to a new disease, and the more it seemed to be about the promotion of a new code of sexual behaviour. Not only were fears being needlessly inflamed, but this was being done to establish new norms of acceptable and appropriate behaviour.

As the Aids panic fluctuated in intensity through the 1990s, it was succeeded by further health scares – from cot death to mad cow disease. It was also supplemented by a systematic government drive to change personal behaviour in areas such as smoking, alcohol, diet and exercise through the 1992 *Health of the Nation* initiative, and by the promotion of mass cancer screening programmes targeted at women (cervical smears and mammograms). To an unprecedented degree, health became *politicised* at a time when the world of politics was itself undergoing a dramatic transformation. The end of the Cold War marked an end to the polarisations between East and West, labour and capital, left and right, that had dominated society for 150 years. The unchallenged ascendancy of the market meant that the scope for politics was increasingly restricted. Collective solutions to social problems had been discredited and there was a general disillusionment with 'grand narratives'. One indication of the resulting ideological and political flux was the fact that the remnants of the left broadly endorsed the Conservative government's Aids campaign (some criticising it for not going far enough), while some right-wingers challenged its scaremongering character (though a few hardliners demanded a more traditional anti-gay, anti-sex line).

As someone who had always identified with the political left, the ending of the old order in the late 1980s led to some contradictory and disconcerting developments. In response to a series of setbacks at home and abroad, the left lowered its horizons and became increasingly moderate and defensive. The weakness of the British left had always been its tendency to confuse state intervention for socialism. In the past, however, the state had intervened in industry and services; now (as it tried to retreat from some of its earlier commitments) it stepped up its interference in personal and family life. The left's endorsement of the government's Aids campaign, following earlier feminist approval of the mass removal of children from parents suspected of sexual abuse in Cleveland, signalled the radical movement's abandonment of its traditional principles of liberty and opposition to state coercion. While most conservative commentators loyally defended government policy, only a small group of free-market radicals was prepared to advance a, rather limited, defence of individual freedom against the authoritarian dynamic revealed in the government's health policies (see Chapter 5).

Until the early 1990s, politics and medical practice were distinct and separate spheres. Some doctors were politically active, but they conducted these activities in parties, campaigns and organisations independent of their clinical work. No doubt, their political outlook influenced their style of practice, but most patients would have scarcely been aware of where to place their doctor on the political spectrum. Systematic government interference in health care has since eroded the boundary between politics and medicine, substantially changing the content of medical practice and creating new divisions among doctors. Thus, for example, the split between fundholding and non-fundholding GPs in the early 1990s loosely reflected party-political allegiances as well as the divide between, on the one hand, suburban and rural practices, and on the other, those in inner cities. Despondent at the wider demise of the left, radical doctors turned towards their workplaces and played an influential role in implementing the agenda of health promotion and disease prevention, and in popularising this approach among younger practitioners. Allowing themselves the occasional flicker of concern at the victimising character of official attempts at lifestyle modification, former radicals reassured themselves with the wishful thinking that it was still possible to turn the sow's ear of coercive health promotion into the silk purse of community empowerment. Reflecting the wider exhaustion of the old order throughout Western society, an older generation of more conservative and traditional practitioners either capitulated to the new style or grumpily took early retirement.

In 1987 I co-authored *The Truth About The Aids Panic*, challenging the way in which the 'tombstones and icebergs' campaign had grossly exaggerated the dangers of HIV infection in Britain, causing public alarm out of all proportion to the real risk (Fitzpatrick, Milligan 1987). Though the central argument of this book was rapidly vindicated by the limited character of the epidemic, it received an overwhelmingly hostile response, particularly from the left. Radical bookshops either refused to stock it or insisted on selling it with an inclusion warning potential readers that it might prove dangerous to their health. In public debates I was accused of encouraging genocide and there were demands that I should be struck off the medical register. My argument that safe sex was simply a new moral code for regulating sexual behaviour provoked particular animosity from those who took the campaign's disavowal of moralism at face value. Not only does moralism not need a dog collar, in the 1990s it was all the more effective for being presented through the medium of the Terrence Higgins Trust, once aptly characterised as the Salvation Army without the brass band.

When the intensely irrational and intemperate climate generated by the Aids panic had abated to some degree in the mid-1990s, I began work on another book (which evolved into this one) aiming to trace the evolution of that scare in the wider political and medical context of the period. Given the pressures of full-time general practice, intensified by the various government reforms and campaigns, this project took rather longer than intended and, in 1996, I applied for a period of study leave. This was rejected by the Department of Health on the grounds that the proposed project was not 'in the interests of medicine in a broad sense or otherwise in the interests of the NHS as a whole'. Whether or not this is so, I now leave to the judgement of my readers.

The fact that I was obliged to carry on working on this project in the interstices of the working day has meant that it has taken rather longer than anticipated. This has, however, enabled me to take into account the accelerated development of some of the trends of the early 1990s in the period since New Labour's electoral triumph in 1997. The scope of government intervention in personal life through the medium of health has expanded – into areas such as domestic violence and parenting – and it has become more authoritarian – notably in the programme for maintaining heroin users on long-term methadone treatment. Yet the remarkable feature of New Labour's public health initiatives is that they have provoked virtually no criticism either from the world of medicine or from that of politics, from any part of the political spectrum. The collapse of both the old left and the new right gives New Labour unprecedented authority to push forward both its authoritarian public health policy and its ill-considered programme of 'modernisation' in the health service. Whatever the fate of Tony Blair's subordination of the NHS to electoral expediency, it is time to expose the deeper processes of the medicalisation of life and the corruption of medicine.

In relation to my earlier dispute with the Department of Health, I would like to acknowledge the support of Diane Abbott, Mildred Blaxter, Gene Feder, Michael Neve, Peter Toon and Tony Stanton. In relation to this book, I am especially grateful to Mary Langan for assistance in many areas and to my medical colleagues Matthew Bench, Tricia Bohn, Gabriella Clouter, Chris Derrett, Janet Williams and Fayez Botros. Thanks are also due to Toby Andrew, Jennifer Cunningham, John Fitzpatrick, Liz Frayn, Heather Gibson, John Gillott, Sally Goble, James Heartfield, Brid Hehir, Gavin Poynter, Mark Wilks. I am particularly thankful to Mick Hume, the courageous editor of LM magazine, where many of the ideas developed here first appeared. I also pay tribute to all the staff and patients at Barton House Health Centre to whom this book is dedicated.

Michael Fitzpatrick
April 2000

GLOSSARY OF ACRONYMS

ADHD	Attention Deficit Hyperactivity Disorder
Aids	Acquired Immune Deficiency Syndrome
ASH	Action on Smoking and Health
BMA	British Medical Association
BMJ	*British Medical Journal*
BSE	Bovine Spongiform Encephalopathy (aka Mad Cow Disease)
CHD	Coronary Heart Disease
CJD	Creutzfeldt-Jakob Disease (also nvCJD: new variant CJD)
CMO	Chief Medical Officer
DHSS	Department of Health and Social Security
DoH	Department of Health
ETS	Environmental Tobacco Smoke (inhaled by passive smokers)
GMC	General Medical Council
GP	General Practitioner
HIV	Human Immunodeficiency Virus
ME	Myalgic Encephalomyelitis (aka Chronic Fatigue Syndrome)
NHS	National Health Service
NICE	National Institute of Clinical Excellence
PHA	Public Health Alliance
RCGP	Royal College of General Practitioners
RCP	Royal College of Physicians
RCPsych	Royal College of Psychiatrists
UNICEF	United Nations Children's Fund
WHO	World Health Organisation

1

INTRODUCTION

We live in strange times. People in Western society live longer and healthier lives than ever before. Yet people seem increasingly preoccupied by their health. There is a widespread conviction that the modern Western diet and lifestyle are uniquely unhealthy and are the main causes of the contemporary epidemics of cancer, heart disease and strokes. The fears provoked and sustained by an apparently endless series of health scares, backed up by government and public health campaigns, tend to encourage a sense of individual responsibility for disease. In exploring these trends, this book seeks to advance what to many will seem a counter-intuitive proposition – that the government's public health policy is really a programme of social control packaged as health promotion. In responding to, and even more by fomenting, increasing public anxiety, the government is seizing the opportunity to introduce a new framework within which people can more comfortably live, so long as they adhere to new rules and accept an unprecedented degree of supervision of their personal lives.

In 1999 the New Labour government in Britain declared its commitment to the promotion of health and the prevention of disease in the White Paper *Saving Lives: Our Healthier Nation* (DoH 1999). The government set targets by which progress could be measured in reducing rates of heart disease and strokes, accidents, cancers and suicides. The public health White Paper put forward a strategy to link national targets to local initiatives, and it outlined plans to pursue health goals in schools, workplaces and neighbourhoods. It aimed to replace exhortations to behave virtuously (stop smoking, curtail drinking, take exercise, eat healthily, etc., etc.) with an effective system for regulating personal behaviour. In this way the government offered the prospect of a longer life – but at the cost of an even more extensive and intrusive system of state regulation of individual behaviour.

Working as a general practitioner, I am struck by the contrast between two types of patient. I see many young people, usually in professional occupations, who worry about their health, watch their diet and take regular exercise. They also seek regular check-ups and screening tests for various diseases. I also see many old people, often former manual workers, who have never been much concerned about their health and have rarely modified their lifestyles or consulted their doctors with a view to preserving it. If you congratulate them on their longevity, they often say that they only wish they had not lived so long. Sometimes they even request my help in assisting their escape from the misery of loneliness, infirmity and poverty. To the former, government health campaigns are a welcome response to a heightened sense of individual vulnerability to environmental dangers. The popular resonance for appeals for greater health awareness reflects the anxieties and insecurities that particularly afflict the younger and more prosperous sections of society. To an older and less affluent generation, these campaigns simply confirm the shift of the health service, as well as other institutions in society, away from any real concern for their needs.

The positive response to official public health documents, such as *Saving Lives* and earlier health promotion initiatives, from the medical profession and the media in general, indicates the widespread acceptance of the basic assumptions of these pro-grammes. But, aside from the specific proposals, some questions arise concerning the underlying principles. We can begin by noting a striking paradox: at a time when, by any objective criterion, people enjoy better health than at any time in human history, the government appears driven to ever greater levels of intervention to improve people's health. Take life expectancy: the commitment to increase it is the first of the 'aims' proclaimed by the White Paper. As this is widely taken as self-evident, it receives no justification. But why should this be the ultimate target of medical science, let alone of government policy, least of all at a time when the increasing longevity of the population has become a widely acknowledged social problem? (Mullan 1999). A boy born in Britain today can expect to live until he is nearly 75; a girl until over 80. Life expectancy has increased by more than 30 years over the past century and by around a decade since the Second World War, apparently without the benefit of government-sanctioned measures of health improvement. It is clear that we have not only exceeded the biblical lifespan of 'three score and ten' but that more and more of us are reaching closer and closer to the biological limit of the human species.

There is much scientific debate about whether further increase in life expectancy is possible. But is it desirable? For many of my patients, the prospect of prolonging their stay in a world that has little time or respect for them has little appeal. The controversy over euthanasia and the romanticisation of suicide among young men (such as rock stars Kurt Cobain and Michael Hutchence) reflect a deeply pessimistic current in contemporary society. The desire simply to live longer by taking health precautions may be interpreted as another way of responding to the perception that life in modern society lacks meaning and purpose. The promoters of health awareness will object that their emphasis is not so much on ensuring that people live longer as on preventing premature deaths. They will point out that, even though there is an average life expectancy of 75–80, more than 90,000 people die every year in the UK before the age of 65. Furthermore, some 32,000 of these deaths are from cancer and 25,000 from heart disease and strokes, many of which could have been prevented. In this context, the concept of prevention is abused: death cannot be prevented, only postponed. Unfortunately, given the current state of medical science, death can generally be postponed only for a relatively short time by relatively intensive preventive measures.

In the nineteenth century, public health measures to improve sanitation and housing played a decisive role in curtailing the epidemics of infectious diseases that devastated the urban poor. Over the past two decades, proponents of the 'new public health' have emphasised the promotion of a healthy lifestyle as the key strategy to combat the modern epidemics of heart disease and cancer. The central weakness of the new public health is the fact that the scope for significant postponement of death from the major causes of premature mortality by preventive measures is limited, though the costs are often substantial. Thus, for example, the increase in average life expectancy to be gained from a 10 per cent reduction in the level of serum cholesterol in the population at large (a much vaunted target of the 1992 *Health of the Nation* White Paper, though dropped in the 1999 document) is between 2.5 and 5 months (Bonneux, Barendregt 1994). However, even to achieve this degree of reduction in cholesterol would require either drastic dietary modification or long-term drug treatment (with its attendant side-effects).

Advocates of the new public health will further object that their aim is not only to increase life expectancy, but also to improve the quality of life, to 'increase the number of years lived free from illness' – in the words of the White Paper. Now it is true that the fact that old people live longer does not necessarily mean that they suffer worse health. However, it is also true that there is a tendency for the prevalence of common chronic degenerative conditions – heart disease, stroke, cancer, osteoarthritis, diabetes, dementia – to increase with age. What is by no means clear is the contribution of the various preventive measures favoured by the government to improving the quality – as distinct from the duration – of people's lives. Indeed it may well be the case that an old person's enjoyment of a cigarette, a cream bun and a bottle of Guinness is more important to them than the extra few weeks they might spend in a life of miserable abstinence.

A further aim of government public health policy is to 'narrow the health gap' between rich and poor by concentrating its efforts on improving the health of the 'worst off in society'. Here is another paradox: the government and the medical profession have become more preoccupied with the relationship between inequality and health at a time when social differentials in health are less significant in real terms than ever before. No doubt it is true that people who are better off are healthier and that the poor are sicker. A vast edifice of epidemiological data has been erected in recent years substantiating these differentials in great detail in relation to every disease and health indicator. Yet the simple contrasts between the health gap that exists in Britain today and that between rich and poor in Victorian England, or that which still prevails between Western and Third World countries today, is enough to expose the lack of historical or social perspective of contemporary public health.

Take infant mortality, one of the most intensively studied indices of population health. The persistent gap between the rate of infant deaths among rich and poor has been a particular focus of the new public health since the publication of the Black Report in 1980 (Black 1980; Townsend, Davidson 1992). The 1990 figures reveal that the number of babies whose fathers are classified as 'unskilled workers' (social class V) who die in the first year of life is 11.7 per 1000 live births, whereas that among the professions (social class I) is 6.2 per 1000 (OPCS 1992). In other words, the infant mortality rate for the poor is nearly twice that among the rich. While there can be little doubt that the persistence of this differential is a

4

pernicious effect of Britain's class divided society, it is important to place it in a wider context. The overall rate of infant deaths in 1990 was slightly less than 8, by 1996 it had fallen below 6. At the turn of the century the figure was around 150, by the Second World War it was still above 50; it did not fall below 20 until the 1960s (Halsey 1988) In some Third World countries today, the infant mortality rate remains comparable with that of Britain in the early decades of this century: for example, India – 94, Bangladesh – 114, Egypt – 61, Mali – 164 (Gray 1993:11). Infant mortality has fallen dramatically among all social classes in Britain in the course of the twentieth century. In 1922 infant mortality among unskilled workers was 97; for the children of professionals, the rate was 38 (Halsey 1988). Over the past 70 years, the rate has fallen to roughly the same extent – between 80 and 90 per cent – among both the richest and the poorest. The infant mortality rate among the poorest families today is similar to that of the richest in the 1970s.

As new public health statisticians are well aware, it is possible, by carefully choosing your starting point and other manoeuvres, to reveal slight increases or decreases in class differentials in infant mortality. But what all such comparisons of mortality rates obscure is the dramatic decline in the absolute number of infant deaths. In 1990 the total number of babies dying in the first year of life in England and Wales was 3,390; in 1900 the figure was 142,912, in 1940 it was still higher by a factor of ten and in 1970 more than four times greater (OPCS 1990; Halsey 1988). The 1990 figure included 248 deaths among babies of parents in social class I and 243 in social class V (though the total number of babies born in this category was half that of class I). Though infant deaths may be relatively more common in poorer families, they are very uncommon in any section of society. A commonplace event within living memory in Britain, the death of an infant has now become a rarity. Furthermore many of these deaths result from conditions such as prematurity and congenital abnormalities, which are often difficult to prevent or treat, or are 'cot deaths', the causes of which are uncertain and preventive measures remain controversial. Again, it seems that the level of government and official medical intervention is out of all proportion to the scale of the problem.

The more closely you examine the new public health the more strange its focus on problems of vanishing significance appears. Yet, despite the limited scope for preventing disease by changing lifestyle, campaigns endorsed by the government and the medical profession to alter individual behaviour have had a major impact on society over the past decade. Nobody capable of watching television can now be in any doubt that smoking cigarettes, drinking alcohol, eating rich food and not taking enough exercise are not good for your health. These basic preoccupations have been supplemented and reinforced by numerous panics about other health dangers from HIV/Aids and BSE/CJD to sunlight, salmonella and listeria.

The expanding range of medical intervention characterised as the *medicalisation* of life involves two inter-related processes. On the one hand, there is a tendency to expand the definition of disease to include a wide range of social and biological phenomena. Thus, for example, while the inclusion of crime within the medical framework remains controversial, the excessive consumption of alcohol or the use of illicit drugs are now widely accepted as medical problems. So too is obesity, a biological variant which is acknowledged as a disease state: by American National Institutes of Health criteria, some two thirds of adult males are affected. According to some criteria, around two-thirds of the British population suffer from a raised cholesterol level (DoH 1992: 56). In a similar way, substantial proportions of the population are arbitrarily designated as having a high blood pressure.

On the other hand, people suffering from this expanded range of disease states are increasingly evaluated in psychological or moral terms. Now that the causes of the old epidemic infectious diseases have largely been discovered and effective treatments developed, they have lost their menace and their mystery. By contrast, the causes of modern epidemics remain obscure and effective cures elusive. Today there is a tendency to believe that people become ill because they want to (as for example in the view that cancer results from 'stress' or depression) or because they deserve to (because they smoke or drink too much). While people who succumb to viruses or bacteria are generally regarded as unfortunate and worthy of sympathy, those who get cancer or heart disease are, at least to a degree, held up to blame for their unhealthy lifestyle. Infection with HIV, though a virus, is ideally suited to the prevailing discourse of individual moral culpability because of its major modes of transmission in Britain – through sex, particularly gay sex, and drug abuse.

If disease is the wages of sin in modern Britain, medicine has become a quasi-religious crusade against the old sins of the flesh. The trend for religion to give way to science and for the scientist to take over the role of the priest has been a feature of modern society since the Enlightenment. The success of scientific medicine in the twentieth century has particularly enhanced the social prestige of the medical profession. Yet it seems that the final triumph of doctors as guardians of public morality comes at a time when they are generally incapable of explaining or curing the major contemporary causes of death and disease.

Successive governments have taken up the issue of health as a convenient vehicle for promoting the gospel of individual responsibility in a period of increasing fragmentation and insecurity. From the late 1970s onwards, advocates of the new public health have promoted the World Health Organisation's definition of health as 'a state of complete physical, mental and social wellbeing' to legitimise the expansion of state medical intervention into wider areas of the life of society (MacKenzie 1946). Though given some impetus by the *Health of the Nation* initiative of the early 1990s, there was always some Conservative reticence about the level of state intervention it demanded. It was not until after the Labour victory in 1997 that the agenda of the new public health could be implemented without restraint.

By the time of the 1998 public health Green Paper, the conception of health put forward by the government seemed to have little to do with disease at all. At the outset it defined good health as 'the foundation of a good life' (DoH February 1998:7). This recalls the classical motto, popularised in the Victorian era – 'a healthy mind in a healthy body' – and establishes a link between physical condition and moral character. It implies that self-discipline and abstinence, the 'mortification of the flesh', can improve the quality of life, in a sense by purifying the soul. Even more insidiously and offensively, it also implies that physical impairment or disease either express or entail moral turpitude, a 'bad' life.

However, by contrast with the Victorian notion of a link between individual fitness and national efficiency, New Labour's interest in health is not inspired by any wider social vision. On the contrary, it reflects the outlook of a society which has abandoned any grand project, in which the horizons of the individual have been reduced to their own body:

> No matter what goes wrong in life – money, work or relationship problems – good health helps sustain us. How often have we all heard somebody say that although things may not be going well – at least they have their health. Good health is treasured.
>
> (DoH February 1998: 7–8)

In this homily, health is reduced to a source of consolation for people who have given up on any higher ambition. In a society of low expectations, the goal of human existence is redefined as the quest to prolong its duration.

Once health is linked with virtue, then the regulation of lifestyle in the name of health becomes a mechanism for deterring vice and for disciplining society as a whole. The new government health policies no longer focus on health in the familiar sense of treating illness and disease, but rather encourage a redefinition of health in terms of the ways in which we live our lives. Under cover of the dubious notion that an extended life (at whatever cost to ourselves and to society) is good for us, the government is providing, and even imposing, its version of the good life. This good life is not simply a longer life, but a longer life lived healthily, which is to say, virtuously. This process is nonetheless insidious for being both well-intentioned and well-supported by many doctors, medical bodies and voluntary organisations. While answering the deep need of some for a framework through which to pull society together in troubled times, for those who are unable or unwilling to respond to the demands of the new public health, it may well be experienced as paternalistic if not overtly oppressive.

One of the few writers to comment on the moralising of disease from a liberal humanist viewpoint is the American critic Susan Sontag. In *Illness as Metaphor*, published in 1978 following her personal experience of cancer, she discussed the way in which the myth of individual responsibility has shifted in modern times from tuberculosis to cancer. In her 1989 sequel, *Aids and its Metaphors*, she noted that the main theme in the response to Aids in the USA is the backlash against the 'permissiveness' of the sixties: 'fear of sexuality is the new, disease-sponsored register of the universe of fear in which everyone now lives' (Sontag 1989: 159). She regretted the impact of the Aids panic in America in both reinforcing moralistic attitudes towards sex and the wider culture of individualism.

Sontag also reflected on the reasons why the Aids panic had such a resonance in modern America. She noted the popularity of apocalyptic scenarios such as nuclear holocaust and ecological catastrophe, reflecting a sense of cultural distress and of society reaching a terminus: 'There is a broad tendency in our culture, an end-of-an-era feeling, that Aids is reinforcing; an exhaustion for many of purely secular ideals' (Sontag 1989: 164). While people with Aids adopted programmes of self-management and self-discipline, diet and exercise, Sontag recognised that the wider Aids panic connected with a public mood of restraint, 'a positive desire for stricter limits on the conduct of personal life', encouraging attitudes such as 'Watch your appetites. Take care of yourself. Don't let yourself go' (Sontag 1989: 163). The prevailing climate of impending doom provided ideal conditions for health scares and for the promotion of virtuous life-styles.

In response to criticisms of the 'victim-blaming' character of much health promotion propaganda, its leading advocates have attempted to soften its individualistic emphasis. Thus the 1998 Green Paper insisted that 'health is not about blame, but about opportunity and responsibility' (DoH February 1998: 28). In the same spirit, the 1999 White Paper *Saving Lives* acknowledged that past health promotion initiatives placed too much emphasis on simply trying to change individual behaviour and explicitly recognised the contribution of the government and local agencies – councils, health authorities, voluntary organisations, businesses – towards achieving targeted improvements in health. However, a glance at the detailed proposals suggests that the opportunities largely fall to the government and local agencies and the responsi-bilites fall on the individual. Where there are opportunities for individuals, these turn out to be opportunities to fulfil responsibilities as defined by the government.

The White Paper elaborates at considerable length the roles of different 'players' in the contract for health. In addition to pro-viding the policy and legislative framework, the government also undertakes to evaluate the health implications of all its policies. Indeed it seems inclined to review its entire programme through the prism of health. Thus, for example, its 'tough measures on crime' may gain in popular approval by being presented as a contribution to public health. For local 'players', collaboration between health and local authorities in 'health action zones' and in the pursuit of 'health improvement programmes' is the central theme. 'Healthy living centres', financed by £300 million from the National Lottery, will seek to 'provide opportunities for local community action to improve health and for individuals to take responsibility for improving their own health' (DoH 1999: 46).

When it comes to the individual there is little left to be said: 'it is finally up to the individual to choose whether to change their behaviour to a healthier one' (DoH February 1998: 48). The vaguely menacing tone is complemented by a reminder that 'individual responsibility is not just about our own health' and a warning about the dangers of passive smoking, setting a bad example to others – particularly by parents to their children. The authoritarian dynamic in New Labour's public health policy becomes increasingly apparent as we move from the discussion of aims and targets to the local 'healthy settings' in which the policy will be implemented and contract compliance enforced. 'The contract will only work if everybody plays their part and everyone is committed to fulfilling their responsibilities' declares the Green Paper in a tone reminiscent of a headteacher's lecture, a managerial pep talk or a vicar's sermon (DoH February 1998: 29). In 'healthy schools', children will have their eating habits monitored to promote 'healthy eating' and be dragooned into physical exercise. Meanwhile in their 'healthy workplaces' their parents will be following the government's list of precise instructions for 'employees'. They can 'play their part in following health and safety guidelines', 'work with employers to create a healthy working environment', 'support colleagues who have problems or who are disabled' and 'contribute to charitable and social work through work-based voluntary organisations' (DoH February 1998: 51).

In my surgery I see two striking consequences of the ascendancy of the new public health. On the one hand, I meet the burgeoning numbers of the 'worried well', young people who would once have been considered healthy, but are now – with official encouragement – anxiously seeking 'check-ups' and advice about an ever widening range of diseases about which there is an ever increasing level of awareness. The facts that many of these diseases are rare, that screening tests are often not helpful and that preventive measures seldom have proven value makes no difference to the demand for advice, assessment or reassurance. On the other hand, I meet many older people with serious health problems caused by osteoarthritis of the hip, cataracts or coronary heart disease who are suffering (and sometimes dying) waiting months and years for surgical treatments. While resources are poured into projects that use health to enhance social control, real health needs – especially those of the elderly – are neglected.

In the following chapters we will be looking more closely at different aspects of the medicalisation of society, including both the widening range of medical intervention and at its greater penetration into the personal life of the individual. This is a process with adverse consequences for the individual and for society. Despite the fact that more people enjoy better health, the intense awareness of health risks means that people feel more ill. This results in an increasing burden of demand on the health care system that every Western society experiences growing difficulty in meeting.

In the penultimate chapter we turn to examine the current crisis of medicine and the medical profession – a set of issues which may appear unconnected to the process of medicalisation. Indeed, early critics of the medicalisation of society depicted this as a process driven by medical authorities and anticipated that it would lead to a further growth in medical prestige and power (Zola 1972). In fact, though, doctors have made a substantial contribution to the medicalisation process, as a profession they can scarcely be regarded today as its beneficiaries. The new millennium finds the medical profession in an unprecedented crisis of confidence, with its leaders expressing a beleagured and inward-looking mentality and its ordinary members preoccupied with stress. Through surveying the evolution of the crisis of medicine we can examine the contribution of both internal factors (the specific difficulties of post-war medical science) and external factors (the influence of the social and political events of recent decades). From this perspective, the trend towards medicalisation may be seen as both a consequence of the wider problems of medicine and as a factor exacerbating them.

The relentless politicisation of health under New Labour, which gathered momentum when the prime minister assumed personal responsiblity for the modernisation of the NHS in early 2000, is destined to intensify the process of medicalisation – and the problems of the medical profession and the health service. The key problem is that, just as the role of medicine in society has expanded, the NHS is called upon to play an ever wider role in the life of the nation. When most other institutions that once inspired popular loyalty are now, like the Royal Family, widely scorned, and attempts to foster a collective spirit around Britpop and the Dome have proved a big disappointment, New Labour is left with that great standby of Old Labour politicians, the 'jewel in the crown' of the post-war welfare state – the NHS.

The NHS serves as a focus for New Labour's populist gestures to the consumer culture which it believes to be the authentic voice of today's Britain: hence NHS Direct and walk-in GP surgeries. It is also a key target of Tony Blair's modernising zeal as he takes on those whom he has designated the 'forces of conservatism' in the crusade for quality, transparency and accountability. The NHS is also expected to help in the government's drive to foster new bonds of community, through encouraging collaboration in the name of health among different agencies and professionals. New Labour hopes to take advantage of the prestige of the NHS to advance its project of revitalising the institutional framework of British society and restoring the links between the individual and the state. Even though the government has allocated more funds to the health service, its wider policies are imposing a burden of expectations that will be almost impossible to fulfil, but will have far reaching consequences for our ability to live our lives as we choose.

2

HEALTH SCARES AND
MORAL PANICS

The Aids panic that took off in the late 1980s and surged through the 1990s was the greatest health-related scare of our time. It had a profound effect on society and accelerated changes in the relationships between the state and the individual, and between doctor and patient, that had been proceeding more gradually over the previous decade. A phenomenon of much wider significance than the novel viral infection on which it was based, the panic was both a product of the peculiar insecurities of the historical moment in which it emerged and a force which intensified them. While the panic provoked private fears of a deadly disease, it also fostered new institutions embodying new forms of solidarity and promoted, in the form of the safe sex code, a new moral framework. It encouraged an already growing preoccupation with health or, to be more precise, with disease. The contemporary obsession with illness and death, with morbidity and mortality, so powerfully reinforced by the Aids crisis, increased the dependence of patient on doctor and strengthened the authority of the state over the individual.

My first encounter with the Aids scare followed the death of Rock Hudson in 1985, before the panic had really taken off. This former matinee idol had died soon after the devastating impact of Aids had led to the public confirmation of both the nature of his illness and his homosexuality. A middle aged woman – a former fan, who had closely followed the news-story – went into a panic attack when she realised that she had shared a coffee cup with a gay man at work and came rushing in to the surgery. I heard several similar stories after the panic proper took off towards the end of 1986, and then again after the death of pop singer Freddie Mercury in 1992, and again with each upswing in the level of popular anxiety. I remember a teenage boy who came in following a series of television programmes designed to boost public awareness. Despite his negligible sexual experience, he was worried he had developed Kaposi's sarcoma, a once-rare skin cancer that now appears in some people with Aids. He reckoned that the red patch on his chest looked exactly like the one exhibited in the cause of public health promotion, by an Aids patient on television. In fact, he had ringworm. I remember too a man in late middle age who was terrified that he might have acquired HIV in the course of a single homosexual experience while in the services during the Second World War. The 'worried well' became a recognised disease category, their anxieties accepted as a price worth paying for heightened Aids awareness.

The Aids panic provided the model for numerous subsequent scares, none reaching the same dimensions, but several making a substantial and enduring impact. Many more minor scares came and went, cumulatively fostering a climate of increasing public anxiety about threats to health that was receptive to a growing scale of state and medical intervention in the personal life of the individual. Alarmed by these scares, people consulted their doctors, not so much because their concern about some particular symptom, but because of their re-interpretation of the significance of this symptom in the light of their new awareness of some wider threat to health. There was (almost) always a rational element in their concern: there was a real threat to health (to some people) at the root of most of the major scares and many of the minor ones. The dominant – irrational – element was expressed in a level of concern that was out of all proportion to the real danger. Let's look at some of the major and minor health scares of the past decade.

Major health scares

HIV/Aids

In November 1986 the British government launched the 'biggest public health campaign in history' about the threat of the Acquired Immune Deficiency Syndrome (Aids) resulting from the Human Immunodeficiency Virus (HIV). Advertisements ominously featuring 'tombstones' and 'icebergs' appeared on television, in cinemas, on high street hoardings and in the press; the 'Don't Die of Ignorance' household leaflet followed in early 1987. The central theme of this campaign was the risk of a major epidemic of HIV disease in Britain resulting from heterosexual transmission. The promotion of 'safe sex' justified by the risk of Aids became the central theme of a barrage of propaganda through the 1990s, with National Aids Day becoming an annual event marked by the wearing of a red ribbon of Aids awareness.

In February 1987 I wrote that there was 'no good evidence that Aids is likely to spread rapidly among heterosexuals in the West', a judgement that has been fully vindicated by subsequent developments (Fitzpatrick, Milligan 1987:8). In 1988 a government working party of top epidemiologists and statisticians predicted that, by 1992, Aids cases would be running at around 3,600 a year, though the press seized on its more alarmist projections that the number of cases could reach 12,000 (DoH 1988). As it turned out, less than 1,500 cases were recorded in 1992. By the end of 1999, some 15 years after the beginning of the epidemic in Britain, the total number of Aids cases had reached around 17,000 (PHLS March 2000). More than two-thirds of these cases were among gay men (who had accounted for almost 90 per cent of cases in the late 1980s). The number of cases spread by drug abusers sharing needles was around 1,000 (a number that had grown much more slowly in the late 1990s). There had been a substantial growth in cases acquired by heterosexual transmission, up to around 3,000, but 2,500 of these had become infected abroad (2,000 in Africa). Of the remainder, less than 300 had become infected through contact with somebody in a recognised high risk group (bisexual/drug user). These figures confirmed as groundless fears that bisexuals and drug users would provide 'a bridge' over which HIV would travel from the recognised high risk groups into the wider heterosexual population.

One small group remained: 252 cases of Aids – in 15 years – in which infection had taken place through heterosexual contact in Britain. Of these 81 had become infected through sex in Britain with somebody who had themselves become infected abroad, outside Europe. The remaining 171 had become infected in Britain through contact with somebody who had become infected in Europe. These 171 cases can be regarded as the central focus of the officially-sponsored Aids panic which was explicitly targeted on the threat of routine heterosexual spread in Britain. Of course the promoters of the panic claim that the fact that this number remained so low confirms the value of their campaign. A more likely explanation is that it confirms that the great heterosexual explosion was never going to happen.

Cot death

In January 1992, following extensive publicity surrounding the cot death of the baby son of television presenter Ann Diamond, the Department of Health launched a national campaign to alert parents to measures they could take to avoid the 'sudden infant death syndrome' (SIDS). The 'Back to Sleep' campaign advised parents to stop smoking, to avoid overheating their babies with blankets and to put them to sleep lying on their backs. This advice followed surveys in New Zealand and Avon which reported fewer deaths from 'sudden infant death syndrome' after such guidelines were introduced. Though campaigners claimed the credit for a subsequent decline in cot deaths, from 1,008 in 1991 to 424 in 1996, this cannot be taken at face value. This rare condition was only recognised as a distinct entity in 1954, in the context of the general decline in infant mortality, and the move towards closer scrutiny of deaths at different stages in the first year of life (Armstrong 1986). A diagnosis of SIDS was only accepted as a cause of death for certification purposes in 1971. The figures vary according to how the condition is defined and rely on the dubious accuracy of death certificates. It has long been recognised that these deaths result from a variety of causes, including a significant, though intensely disputed, proportion from infanticide (Green 1999; Meadow 1999; Emery, Waite 2000). There is no explanation for the danger to babies of sleeping on their front and it seems a highly improbable cause of death. This theory also fails to explain apparent seasonal variations in cot death and the significantly higher incidence among boys. Another theory – that cot deaths resulted from the inhalation of toxic fumes arising from chemicals applied to babies' mattresses – enjoyed a brief flurry of publicity before being discredited (Limerick 1998).

The main effect of the cot death campaign was to raise parental awareness of a rare condition and to intensify their anxieties about their babies' health. I have talked to several parents who have watched their babies through the night, carefully turning them over on to their backs whenever they rolled over, lest they find them dead in the morning. I have not met parents whose smoking has been blamed for their baby's death, but the cot death campaign must have compounded their feelings of guilt and pain.

Malignant moles

Health promotion around the link between exposure to sunlight and skin cancer gathered momentum through the 1990s (Fitzpatrick, Hehir 1999). In 1995 the Health Education Authority launched its 'Sun know how' campaign, followed up in 1996 with the slogan 'Shift to the shade'. The Australian advice 'slip, slap, slop' – slip on a shirt, slap on a hat, slop on some suncream – has been widely adopted as part of the sun awareness crusade in Britain. Schools have been a particular target as children are advised to play in shaded areas, wear Legionnaire-style hats and long-sleeved shirts. 'Molewatch' teams patrol beaches in seaside resorts urging holiday-makers to cover up their dangerously exposed skin.

Though public anxieties are focused on malignant melanoma – moles which turn cancerous – in fact these are a relatively rare type of skin cancer and the one least related to sunlight. They account for less than 10 per cent of skin cancers, around 4,000 cases a year in Britain. These commonly arise in areas of the body not much exposed to the sun, such as the back of the legs, soles of the feet, scalp and buttocks and they are as common in Japan, where sunbathing is not customary, as they are in the West. Though if diagnosed early and treated aggressively, most are curable, some cases are highly malignant and spread early to other parts of the body, resulting in a significant mortality (around 1,500 deaths a year). According to Newcastle dermatologist Sam Shuster, the dramatic increase in the number of 'suspicious' moles removed and sent for microscopic examination over the past decade has been paralleled by a tendency to reclassify benign disease as malignant (Shuster 1992). His conclusion is that 'melanomas are being invented, not found' and that the resulting 'spurious cures' are being 'used to justify an incompetent and frightening screening programme'. Shuster's colleague, Jonathan Rees believes that there is 'no robust evidence to defend most health promotion in this area' (Rees 1996).

The Pill

In October 1995 the government's Committee on the Safety of Medicines wrote to all doctors and pharmacists alerting them to the dangers of an increased risk of blood clotting disorders (venous thromboembolism) associated with seven named brands of contraceptive pills. These, so-called 'third generation' pills had been introduced in the 1980s because they had a lower incidence of side-effects than earlier preparations. It subsequently emerged that, though there was an increase in the relative risk of these pills, compared with earlier pills, the risk was still half of that of thrombosis in pregnancy. In absolute terms, the risk of dying from thrombosis in any of these circumstances in any one year was around one-third of that involved in playing football (3 fatalities per 100,000). My dominant memory of this scare was of a twenty minute discussion about the different risks of different pills with a young woman, who then announced that she smoked twenty cigarettes a day (which is around two hundred times more of a threat to life than any contraceptive pill).

The immediate consequence of the pill scare was that many women either stopped using the pill or switched to alternative – less effective – methods of contraception. The slightly longer-term consequence was an increase in pregnancies, resulting, according to an authoritative estimate, in around 12,400 additional births and 13,600 additional abortions in 1996 (Furedi 1999). The resulting extra expenditure on maternity and abortion provision was estimated at a total of £67 million.

The 'human form of mad cow disease'

In March 1996, health secretary Stephen Dorrell announced in parliament that, in the absence of any alternative explanation, the most likely cause of the first ten cases of what became known as 'new variant' Creuzfeldt Jakob Disease (nvCJD) was exposure to beef products contaminated with Bovine Spongiform Encephalopathy (BSE) (Fitzpatrick 1998). This announcement had no public health value: measures to prevent transmission of BSE to humans had already been introduced in 1988–89. However, the announcement provoked a spate of 'Mad Cow Can Kill' headlines and a public panic. Beef sales, to the public and to fast food chains, schools and other public institutions plummeted and, within days, the European Union and other overseas importers banned British beef. The consequences for farmers, rapidly pushed into a mass slaughter of herds, and workers in food processing and retailing, were catastrophic. Within twelve months the costs of compensating farmers for their losses passed £3billion.

The number of cases of nvCJD grew slowly, to reach a total of around fifty by the end of 1999. Though research suggested some link between BSE and nvCJD, the nature of the connection and, in particular, the mode of transmission remained obscure. Intensive study of each new case failed to reveal any explanation, though the small numbers – and the fact that some of the cases were in long-standing vegetarians – told against any simple spread through eating beef or beef products. Nevertheless many people changed their eating habits lest they succumb to this lethal condition; a few still refuse to take medication in the form of capsules because of their fear of acquiring nvCJD via gelatin.

MMR and autism

In April 1998, gastroenterologist Andrew Wakefield and his colleagues at the Royal Free Hospital in London published a paper claiming to have established a link between the Measles, Mumps and Rubella (MMR) vaccine and autism, through the medium of inflammatory bowel disease (Wakefield *et al.* 1998). They believe that toxins leak through an inflamed bowel wall into the blood stream, leading to the familiar neuro-psychiatric features of autism. This paper and ensuing controversy caused great anxiety among parents whose children were due to have the MMR – and consider-able apprehension among those whose children had recently had it. Many parents of children diagnosed as autistic over the past decade reviewed their child's records in search of any correlation between vaccination and the onset of autistic symptoms.

Though plausible, there was little evidence to support the MMR–autism link (Taylor *et al.* 1999). The theory could not explain why, in the children in the study, autistic behavioural features appeared to predate the bowel inflammation which was supposed to release the toxins. Nor was it possible to show a clear relationship between the vaccination and the onset of autism. This is difficult because, while the MMR immunisation is a fixed event, the emergence of autism is, characteristically, an insidious process whose features become clear over months rather than weeks or days. It has long been recognised that, while some cases of autism are apparent from early infancy, many only become apparent at 18 months or later – shortly after the usual time the MMR is given. It is unlikely that anybody who was not already suspicious that immunisation might be harmful would suspect a link.

The MMR scare led to a period of intensive and prolonged discussions in the baby clinic as parents agonised over the decision whether to have their baby vaccinated, baffled and confused by contradictory medical opinions. It has led inevitably to a fall in the uptake of the vaccine, raising fears of a return of measles if the general level of immunity in the community fell any lower.

Minor health scares

Health scares have something in common with showbiz celebrities, both owing much to the media. Some appear suddenly and after their 'fifteen minutes of fame' disappear as rapidly; others emerge more gradually and remain on the stage for years, though largely in the background; others still have an initial flurry in the limelight, then fade for a while, only to make periodic comebacks before slowly fading. Here is a far from exhaustive list of scares which have one common feature: they have all been raised in one form or another by patients in my surgery over the past decade.

- In May 1994 the country was gripped by fears about *necrotising fasciitis*, a fearsome 'flesh-eating bug' that was ravaging hospital patients, though this turned out to be the haemolytic streptococcus bacterium, a familiar and usually easily treatable pathogen that occasionally causes a fulminating infection in debilitated patients.

- Discussion of the problem of bacterial resistance to antibiotics, a recurrent theme of medical conferences and journals (notably concerns about hospital-acquired Methicillin Resistant Staphylococcus Areus, MRSA, and multi-drug resistant tuberculosis) has spilled over into the popular media, with headlines about *superbugs*, causing anxieties that familiar antibiotics will no longer be effective.

- *Electromagnetic fields (EMF)*, arising from overhead power cables and pylons, or from mobile phones and microwave ovens, have been blamed for brain tumours and other malignancies (though intensive researches have failed to confirm any link).

- An alleged link between *silicone* breast implants and various connective tissue disorders led to a number of high-profile court cases; though authoritative studies failed to substantiate this link, the publicity caused great distress to one patient of mine who had a silicone implant following surgery for breast cancer.

- The threat of *nuclear radiation* became a major public concern after the fire at the Chernobyl power station in the Ukraine in 1986, fuelling continuing speculation about clusters of cases of leukemia in the vicinity of nuclear plants in Britain. In the event, fears of an upsurge in malignancies resulting from Chernobyl were not realised and the theory about leukemia clusters has not been substantiated.

- In December 1988 junior health minister Edwina Currie declared that most of the country's eggs were contaminated with *salmonella*, in a nineteen word statement that cost the government £70 million in compensation to farmers and Mrs Currie her job (North, Gorman 1990). Ten years later an outbreak of gastroenteritis traced to beef contaminated with *E.coli O157* supplied by a Glasgow butcher caused a number of deaths among old people. The fear of lethal infection was added to existing concerns about *food* safety, arising from the use of pesticides on plants, antibiotics and other drugs on animals and diverse additives and preservatives.

- *Water* has also come to be regarded as a source of danger, as a result of *nitrates* derived from fertilisers, or from *toxic wastes* or bacterial contamination (LeFanu 1994). The main consequence is a flourishing trade in bottled water, though this also became the focus of a scare when contaminated stocks provided by a leading supplier had to be removed from supermarket shelves. Signs around canals and waterways warning of the danger of *Weil's disease*, a rare infection transmitted by the urine of rats and almost exclusively affecting sewage workers, have led to at least two requests for blood tests in my surgery.

- The *air* is another source of danger – from atmospheric pollution resulting, in particular, from car exhaust fumes carrying *lead, carbon monoxide* and other toxic chemicals. The air also carries diverse *allergens*, generated by farming (e.g. oil seed rape) and by industrial processes.

Perhaps the greatest irony of the recent wave of scares is that they have taken off at a time when everyday life in Western society is safer than ever and when the quality of our environment and of our food, water and air is higher and more highly regulated than at any time in history.

Scare states

Though health scares may affect anybody, some are more vulnerable than others.

- *Women* are susceptible to campaigns to raise awareness about breast and cervical cancer – and to scares about the inadequacies of screening tests and treatment programmes. Contraception is risky, but so is unprotected sex and the menopause only brings the choice between worrying about osteoporosis and fractures or the side-effects of HRT.

- *Pregnant women* are, according to a cheerful Department of Health pamphlet distributed free of charge at antenatal clinics, at risk from listeria (cheese), toxoplasma (cats), salmonella (eggs), and chlamydia (sheep) (DoH 1991a). In the context of detailed advice on how to avoid these terrifying infections, the pamphlet's comment that they are all 'very rare, and it is unlikely that you or your baby will be affected' is scarcely reassuring. Expectant mothers are also menaced by smoking, drinking and by VDUs.

- *Babies and children* are not only at risk of cot death, immunisation complications and skin damage from sunlight, they are also in danger from 'poisonous dummies' (phthalates), dangerous toys and contaminated baby foods (Durodie 1999). While 'breast is best' and formula feeds potentially harmful, breast milk has also been shown to transmit numerous toxins. The spectre of meningitis, a rare condition whose features are now familiar to millions, hovers over every viral illness which produces a fever and a rash.

- *Men* too are at risk! Jealous at having been left out of earlier health scares, advocates of men's health have tried to catch up by promoting anxieties about prostate and testicular cancer as well as concerns about falling sperm counts.

Key features

A number of common features emerge from our brief survey of some of the more significant health scares of the past decade. At the source of each lies a serious disease, often with a powerful symbolic character. The risk to any particular individual of acquiring this disease may be low, but it is often also either indeterminate or difficult to establish with any accuracy, creating great scope for speculations which invariably feature worst-case scenarios. Though there have been scares in the past, the recent wave is unique in its scope and impact. Let's take these points in turn.

The diseases at the root of the major scares are generally terrifying and often rapidly fatal. Some are grossly debilitating (Aids, nvCJD), others disfiguring (malignant melanoma). Some cause sudden death in previously healthy individuals (cot death in babies, pulmonary embolism in women on the Pill), others cause lifelong disability (autism). All these conditions are difficult, if not impossible, to treat. They often appear to strike the most vulnerable, or even if that is not generally the case, as with Aids, 'innocent victims' – babies infected by their mothers, or recipients of infected blood transfusions – are singled out for particular sympathy. Health scares are all the more frightening when they are associated with some intimate or familiar activity, like sex, eating, sunbathing, putting the baby to bed. The apparently random way in which these demons strike, reinforced by the vogue for quoting risks like gambling odds, encourages gloomy forebodings and reinforces a fatalistic outlook.

Health ministers and medical authorities have been criticised for their failings in communicating the subtleties of risk to the public – and thereby inflaming public fears, particularly in relation to mad cow disease and the Pill. No doubt there are real problems here. In the case of the Pill, the risks are so low that they are difficult to measure and, once measured in large population surveys, it is difficult to distinguish between an increase that is statistically significant and one that is significant in terms of clinical practice. In some cases, for example that of the risk of acquiring nvCJD from eating beef, or that of a child becoming autistic as a result of the MMR vaccine, the risk is impossible to quantify (it may well be non-existent). This has led to the absurd demand from campaigners for proof that there is no risk from beef or the MMR vaccine before they can consider it safe for people to be exposed to these potential sources of disease. The very indeterminacy of the risks involved in most health scares allows those who are so inclined to speculate wildly, thus inflating anxieties further and justifying further official intervention.

In the not so distant past the common focus of health scares was the threat of outbreaks of infectious epidemics, which produced demands for quarantine and other restrictions on trade and travel. But, though popular fears of plague and cholera, typhus and typhoid, were intense and often resulted in social and political strife, they were more episodic and more localised than the recent scares. In more recent years, most notably in the USA, there have been health scares about numerous environmental pollutants, from the 'Great Cranberry Juice Scare' of 1959 to the 'Alar and Apples Scare' of 1989, mostly, like these two, of dubious validity (Wildavsky 1995). In Britain, since the 1970s we have had scares about the whooping cough vaccine, about tampons causing 'toxic shock syndrome' and about the side-effects of various drugs. Yet there are two key differences between the scares of the late 1980s and 1990s and those of earlier years. First, whereas the response of the government and medical authorities in the past was generally to try to dampen public fears and to assuage anxieties, now we are more likely to find politicians and medical experts initiating, if not actively promoting, health scares. (Though scares about the Pill and BSE originated in government committees, they erupted out of control, causing unpredicted and undesired consequences. The MMR–autism scare is the only major scare which the authorities seriously attempted to discourage, fearing the consequences for the entire child immunisation programme.) Second, the public today is much more engaged in controversies around health issues and is much more responsive to health scare campaigns. The result is that health scares have acquired a virtually continuous presence in the life of society, coexisting with a unprecedented level of free-floating anxiety about health, which may focus for a shorter or longer period on one particular scare, before moving on to the next.

Impact

It is possible to identify four stages through which health scares pass, at different rates and different levels of intensity.

1 Build-up

Major health scares rarely appear without advance warning, as they have usually been developing gradually over a period of some years. In some cases there is what appears in retrospect as an anticipatory phase: thus the herpes scare of the early 1980s in many ways foreshadowed the Aids panic. Among the few beneficiaries of Aids (apart from those in the booming business of health promotion)

were people with herpes, for whom all manner of grim consequences had been predicted as a result of life-long infection and
frequent recurrences, all of which were forgotten when the more
potent menace of HIV emerged. In relation to other scares there
were earlier minor outbreaks – such as the links between the Pill
and breast cancer – which prepared the way for the big one.
Rumbling anxieties about childhood immunisations had continued
since the whooping cough scare of the 1970s, despite studies which
failed to confirm the alleged link to brain damage. Yet a vague
popular awareness of these controversies, assiduously encouraged
by anti-immunisation pressure groups, ensured that there was a
ready response to any hint of a problem with MMR.

In the build-up to a health scare, controversies which were
formerly confined to the specialist medical domain begin to spill
over, first into the mainstream medical journals, then into the wider
media. This spill over usually appears at first in the broadsheet
newspapers rather than the tabloids and in science rather than
current affairs or consumer programmes on television. The build up
of a scare is sometimes facilitated by a dissident medical activist or
other campaigner whose challenge to the mainstream consensus
also begins to extend from the professional into the popular
domain. The role of the maverick microbiologist Richard Lacey,
who demanded drastic measures to prevent the spread of BSE to
humans more than five years before the government's announcement that some such link was possible, is one example. Ann
Diamond's campaign around cot death is another, this time led
from inside the media.

2 Take-off

In relation to most major scares, it is possible to define a moment
when they 'went critical' and leapt to the centre of the mass media
and thereby to public attention. If we look at our list, it is striking
that this moment was usually defined by an official government
announcment or political initiative: the 'tombstones and icebergs'
campaign (Aids), the Committee on Safety of Medicine's announcement (the Pill), the Stephen Dorrell statement (BSE–nvCJD).
Alternatively, the take-off was triggered by the appearance of a
report in a prestigious medical journal (MMR-autism). Once these
scares had received an official medical/political launch, the press
and television enthusiastically took them up and transmitted them
to a public with an apparently insatiable appetite for such stories.

Once in the public domain, the scares developed a life of their own, often producing effects far greater than were either expected or desired by their originators, a trend best exemplified by the mad cow panic of 1996.

3 Backlash

At a certain stage, every health scare provokes a critical response towards which there are a number of contributory factors. The backlash usually starts from representatives of a body of medical or scientific opinion which is sceptical of the basis on which the scare has been launched. The challenge to the role of HIV in Aids from the retrovirologist Peter Duesberg and others, together with criticisms of the official line of exaggerating the risk to heterosexuals, provoked some wider questioning of the Aids panic in the early 1990s. In relation to cot death and malignant melanoma, we have already quoted dissident paediatricians and dermatologists. The scares about the Pill and the MMR vaccine were unusual in that most experts in both fields were bemused by the scares from the outset. In the case of the Pill, most family planning authorities did not believe that the reports of increased risk were clinically significant, and in the case of the MMR vaccine, neither gastroenterologists nor child psychiatrists were, in general, much impressed by the evidence adduced by Wakefield and his colleagues. Doubts about the BSE–nvCJD link were even more profound, as the prion theory on which the whole concept of 'transmissible spongiform encephalopathies' is based remains controversial, and various alternative hypotheses concerning the aetiology of these conditions are in circulation.

The media, always alert to a new angle, and particularly keen on controversy, soon pick up the views of critical experts and provide them with a platform from which to expound their views. To some extent the resulting debate helps to keep the panic alive when the public may be beginning to tire of the same old scare story. However, at the same time, it begins to cause some irritation as people become confused by rival arguments, often of an increasingly esoteric character. The popular view that 'if the experts can't agree about these problems, how are we supposed to make up our minds?' adds cynicism to anxiety.

4 *Steady state*

Observers of the recurrent health scares of the past decade sometimes conclude that the public has become so cynical about them that they no longer have much impact. This is seriously to overestimate the scale of the backlash and to underestimate the extent to which even the most sceptical individuals have discreetly modified their lifestyles as a result of the anxieties generated by these scares. As the reactive character of the term backlash implies, it is more of an expression of anger than a systematic attempt to roll back the influence of the phenomenon against which it is reacting. If you examine the influence of any of the major scares we have listed, taking account of the backlash that followed the initial impact, you find that, far from being neutralised by the backlash, the scare continues to have a significant effect, perhaps less than at its peak, but substantial nonetheless. The most obvious example of this is the Aids panic, which has seen off Duesberg and the other dissidents and continues to exert a powerful influence. Perhaps even more significant is the on-going effect of the Pill and MMR scares: even though it emerged that the balance of medical authority was strongly opposed to both scares, the number of women on 'third generation' pills five years later remains substantially reduced and the uptake of the MMR vaccine has yet to reach its pre-scare level.

Once a health scare has established a particular fear in the popular consciousness it can readily be re-activated, either as a matter of deliberate policy or as result of some incident. Thus, for example, in 1999 the government launched a programme for routine testing all pregnant women for HIV. Official statistics show that in 1997 there were 265 births in Britain to women infected with HIV, producing 71 HIV positive babies. These figures are low, and declining, and the vast majority are to be found among refugees from Africa living in London. Irrational from a public health point of view, the universal screening policy was, according to one critic, 'a useful re-affirmation of the politically correct, if not factually correct, mantra that we are all of us at risk of HIV and had better behave with appropriate sexual and social caution' (Bradley 1999). The re-appearance of the sun every spring provides the occasion for a booster of the skin cancer scare. Scares without a seasonal component are obliged to rely on events such as a celebrity death or fall back on the artificial annual 'national awareness' day (or week).

For many, if not most, people life will never be the same as it was before the great health scares of the 1990s. It is, of course, still possible to have sex without using a condom, but as numerous

27

patients have told me, it is not easy to remove from the back of the mind the worry that this might result in a lethal contamination. It is no longer possible to put a baby in a cot without thinking about which way around they should be lying, and without the occasional shiver running down the spine at the thought that they might not survive the night. People still lie in the sun on those rare occasions it appears in Britain's cloudy skies, but usually not without applying their sunscreen cream (even if they do not consult the daily Solar UV Index, and adjust their cream and exposure time according to their skin type, as the summer 1999 official campaign advised). Scarcely a week goes by without somebody asking me whether some harmless mole or minor skin blemish is the first sign of a malignant melanoma (in the ten years I have been running a minor surgery clinic, I have seen only two). Women still take the Pill, but now in a state of heightened awareness of a risk of sudden death from thrombosis that is much less than that of dying in a road accident. The proportion of meat eaters has never returned to the level before the mad cow scare, but even a lifetime of vegetarianism cannot be guaranteed to protect you from nvCJD. Most parents still choose to have their babies vaccinated against measles, mumps and rubella, but none now without a twinge of anxiety that this may destine them to a devastating disability.

When it comes to health scares, everybody has their weak point. People who were fiercely critical of the government's 1998 ban on 'beef-on-the-bone', because of a notional risk of transmission of BSE, may well endorse the government's cot death campaign or refuse to take their child for the MMR vaccine. Others who reject the major scares may find themselves in the grip of the panic over mobile phones or microwaves. Everybody is now more careful about what they eat or drink, more reluctant to take medication, more aware of the need to take precautions against pathogenic forces, of whose existence they were unaware only a few years ago. Whatever their individual proclivities and prejudices, nobody is immune from the consequences of more than a decade of health scares.

Who's to blame?

Doctors overwhelmed by an influx of patients in the grip of the latest health scare usually blame 'the media' for inflaming anxieties with 'sensational' headlines and 'scaremongering' television documentaries. Politicians complain of public complacency if people appear not to follow government health warnings and of over-reaction if they panic and, for example, suddenly refuse to buy British beef. Surveying the damage wrought on British agriculture – and the balance of trade – a week after his parliamentary statement on the supposed BSE–nvCJD link, health minister Stephen Dorrell declared in exasperation in a Radio Four interview that 'it's not the cows that are mad, it's the public' (quoted in Lang 1998). But the mad cow panic did not begin on the farms or in the butchers' shops or supermarkets. It began among the scientists, spread to the politicians and was amplified in their interactions with the media, which transmitted it to the public. Nobody was better placed to dampen down the panic than Dorrell, yet his statement served only to exacerbate the anxieties that devastated farmers in Britain and beyond.

The history of the major scares confirms that they did not originate in spontaneous outbreaks of public anxiety. They each started among doctors and scientists who themselves became alarmed, either at the emergence of a new disease (Aids, nvCJD), or the recognition of a new risk factor (front sleeping, MMR, the Pill). In the absence of any effective treatment for any of these conditions, doctors sought to raise public awareness of them, in the belief that this was the only means of prevention. The scares took off when doctors' own anxieties led them to turn to their contacts with government and the media to generate wider publicity around the focus of their concerns.

A number of factors have encouraged medical and scientific experts to project their anxieties into the public realm. One is the wider crisis of medical confidence in tackling the 'modern epidemics' of coronary heart disease and cancer, now that the threat of infectious diseases has receded. In the 1970s and 1980s, the recognition that effective treatments for these conditions remained elusive led to a swing towards health promotion in the cause of prevention, the subject of the next two chapters. The emergence of Aids, ironically an infectious disease, but one for which neither vaccine nor treatment appeared likely to emerge in the near future, struck terror into the hearts of doctors throughout the West. Their immediate response was to put their hopes in raising public awareness of the danger of epidemic transmission. In the case of Aids in Britain, given the low incidence of HIV infection in the late 1980s, the fact that it is a fragile virus that is fairly difficult to transmit, and given also that it remained virtually exclusive to clearly defined high-risk populations, the risks of a major epidemic were negligible. However, the medical establishment's anxieties about Aids, transmitted to the government, contributed to an official campaign that grossly exaggerated public risks and thereby exacerbated popular anxieties.

The unfolding mad cow panic revealed the increasing irrationality of expert advice to the government and its consequences. When in early 1996, after some years of dismissing suggestions of a link between BSE and CJD, the scientists first noticed a handful of cases that raised this as a real possibility, they were understandably rattled. But instead of calming them down and encouraging further research, ministers themselves panicked and made dramatic public statements which did nothing to reduce risk, but had the effect of inducing mass anxiety and causing the collapse of the beef trade. In December 1997, some twenty months after the initial panic, the government's committee of scientific and medical experts discussed a preliminary report of research which suggested the remote possibility that BSE could be transmitted in dorsal root ganglia (tiny knots of nerve tissue close to the spinal cord) of cattle slaughtered for consumption as beef (Fitzpatrick February 1998) The report estimated that in 1997 some six infected animals might get through the system, and in 1998 possibly three (out of more than two million cattle slaughtered). The committee noted that before the system was tightened up in 1988–89, the figure was many thousand times greater. In response to the expert advice that emerged from these deliberations, the government immediately banned the sale of 'beef on the bone' (which might contain a microscopic amount of BSE infectivity in its dorsal root ganglia), though we were all eating BSE-infected beef by the plateful in the late 1980s (which may or may not have been a factor in the twenty-three cases of nvCJD which had been identified up to the end of 1997). The interaction between scientists and politicians appeared to amplify insecurities on both sides, leading to policy of increasing absurdity.

The role of the media in relation to all the major health scares, and most of the minor ones, has been secondary to that of the medical and political authorities. In the past, investigative journalists have exposed the dangers of medical treatments, such as Thalidomide in the 1960s and the Dalkon shield, an intra-uterine contraceptive device (coil), in the 1970s. It is, however, difficult to think of a more recent example. Recent health scares usually emanate from official – medical, scientific, government – sources, and are amplified by news media which are sensitive to the public resonance for such stories. Far from being critical of the medical and political establishments, media coverage of most of the major scares has been strikingly subservient to the official agenda. In relation to the HIV/Aids panic in particular, the overwhelming bulk of the vast journalistic output has been dedicated to amplifying the themes proclaimed by health ministers and their prominent medical advisers. Indeed when critical articles have appeared, these have been either attacks on the government for not promoting the panic vigorously enough, or directed against critics of the official line like Duesberg, who have been characterised, in a revealing choice of metaphor, as 'Aids heretics'. In some recent cases, such as MMR–autism, silicone implants, Gulf War syndrome, scares have been encouraged by lawyers pursuing 'class actions' in pursuit of compensation for illnesses alleged to result from diverse toxins.

Though the public cannot be fairly blamed for initiating health scares, its ready response certainly revealed a predisposition to panic. The popular appetite for health scare stories and the generally postive public response to related government health promotion initiatives indicated a climate of opinion that was both vulnerable to health-related anxieties and sympathetic to official intervention in the cause of curtailing threats to health.

The role of government

Up to the late 1980s (with the exception of wartime) governments in Britain have always been reluctant to interfere in the personal behaviour of citizens, even in the cause of improving health. This reluctance can be traced back to nineteenth-century traditions of liberal resistance to quarantines and other measures of state repression to prevent the spread of infectious epidemics. Such policies were favoured by the absolutist dictatorships on the European continent, but were regarded as anathema to capitalist principles of individual freedom (especially in matters of trade). Yet these traditions were cast aside in the great health scares of the last decade, in the government's quest for enhanced popularity and authority.

In the run up to the 1982 Conservative Party conference, Mrs Thatcher was obliged to reassure the public that 'the NHS is safe with us', following the leak of proposals for privatisation of health care drawn up by an influential right-wing think tank (Timmins 1995: 393). This statement indicated that, even at the height of her power, Mrs Thatcher could be put on the defensive over health, an issue that had been regarded as the property of the Labour Party since the establishment of the post-war welfare state. Ten years later, Mrs Thatcher's successor, John Major, presided over the launch of *The Health of the Nation*, the most extensive programme of state intervention in personal 'health-related' behaviour ever introduced by any British government – before the public health policies of New Labour after 1997. One of the main forces driving this dramatically rising profile of government intervention in personal health over this period was the parallel decline in the prestige of government. This problem became particularly apparent for Mrs Thatcher in her third term after 1987, when her earlier successes over the unions could no longer compensate for the wider exhaustion of policy that was exposed when the illusion of 'popular capitalism' built on the speculative Thatcher/Lawson boom of the late 1980s was exposed in a new recession. From raising awareness about Aids to preventing heart disease and cancer, campaigning to improve the nation's health offered the government a new vehicle for recovering popular support.

The government also recognised that it was not the only public institution that had suffered a loss of esteem in the eyes of the nation. It was concerned about the decline in influence of traditional sources of authority, such as the mainstream churches, even political parties and trade unions, and the resulting loss of cohesion in society, a trend exacerbated by the increasing economic and social instability of the 1980s. The ready audience for health scares indicated the extent of the process of fragmentation; it also suggested that health might provide a means of official intervention, seeking both to replace defunct mechanisms of regulating personal behaviour and to provide new modes of solidarity.

The Aids panic marked a decisive shift in government policy towards direct intervention in intimate personal behaviour. This shift was all the more significant in that it took place under Mrs Thatcher, who was well-known for her hostility towards state intervention and for her distaste for public discussions about sex. However, though Mrs Thatcher distanced herself personally from the Aids campaign – conspicuously vetoing government support for a proposed national study of sexual habits – she nevertheless made sure that from the outset the campaign was supervised by a top level Cabinet committee. In fact, the Aids campaign was quite compatible with the moralising themes that ran through the Conservative governments of the 1980s and 1990s, from Mrs Thatcher's 'Victorian values' to Mr Major's 'back to basics'. Indeed, because it was more subtle than these campaigns, and organised around an issue of health, the Aids scare proved a vastly more successful moral crusade than these more traditional initiatives.

The key to the success of the moral dimension of the Aids panic was the early shift away from an old-time-religion, explicitly anti-gay, pro-family, approach, which was favoured by some influential clerics, police chiefs and Tory politicians. This outlook, associated with the religious right, remained a persistent, but marginal influence on Aids policy in Britain (though it was more powerful in the USA). By the time the government launched the major Aids campaign in Britain, the distinguishing feature of its morality was its denial of having a moral line. Instead it proclaimed an explicitly non-judgemental, tolerant and pluralistic outlook. The campaign implicitly accepted homosexuality ('gay or straight', as the government's propaganda put it, implying a moral equivalence that was anathema to the Christian right). It also accepted sex outside marriage, another unprecedented public gesture for a Conservative government. In the early stages of the Aids campaign, journalists were bemused to discover that cabinet ministers and senior civil servants were discussing the relative risks of vaginal and anal intercourse, the virtues of oral sex and the delights of condoms; within months these topics had moved to the mainstream media and before long were on the national curriculum.

While radicals and gay activists applauded the government for its boldness in promoting open discussion about matters of sex and urged it to go further, they ignored the fact that the 'safe sex' code promoted by the Aids campaign simply replaced the traditional moral framework with a new one. It replaced the fear of eternal damnation, which no longer offered much of a deterrent to youthful sexual experimentation, with fear of a lethal disease, a much more potent force. The new moral code no longer exhorted people towards 'goodness', but replaced this with the ethic of 'safety', according to which all manner of sexual activity could be classified as 'low', 'medium' or 'high risk'.

Instruction in the new moral framework was provided by an army of Aids activists, employed at every level in health, education, local government as well as through television programmes, posters, leaflets, pamphlets and books. 'Not since the heyday of the Catholic convent school had children been so bluntly instructed in the causal link between sex and terror', wrote Mark Lawson in a retrospective commentary on the Aids campaign in the *Guardian* in 1996 (Lawson 1996). This should not be understood as a critical comment, but as a measure of Lawson's approval. This article was prompted by the revelation that the government had grossly exaggerated the risk of the heterosexual spread of Aids as a way of discouraging young people from having sex. 'The government has lied, and I am glad' was Lawson's opening sentence. He accepted that the government's campaign was based on an 'untruth', but argued that this was a 'good lie', because it had 'spent a huge amount of money ... encouraging reflection and discrimination in the area of sexual behaviour'. This liberal endorsement of the cynical manipulation of public fears of a terrifying, but mercifully rare disease, in the cause of promoting a new framework of sexual morality well sums up the cynical character of the Aids scare and the real moral corruption that it embodied – in medicine as well as in politics and journalism.

3

THE REGULATION OF
LIFESTYLE

Everybody should try to look to after themselves better, by
not smoking, taking more exercise, eating and drinking
sensibly.
(*Saving Lives: Our Healthier Nation*, White Paper
on public health, July 1999, vii)

While clinical trials have shown the benefits of stopping
cigarette smoking, many of the changes in lifestyle that are
being promoted by Western governments are based on information lacking in solid evidence. It is unpardonable to
try to alter the diet of an entire population without sufficient information.
(David Weatherall, *Science and the Quiet Art*, 1995: 311)

Nor can very much be changed by the trendy fashions in
changing 'life-styles', all the magazine articles to the contrary; dieting, jogging, and thinking different thoughts may
make us feel better while we are in good health, but they
will not change the incidence or outcome of most of our
real calamities.
(Lewis Thomas, *The Fragile Species*, 1992: 14–15)

David Weatherall, currently director of the Institute of Molecular
Medicine at Oxford, and formerly Nuffield professor of clinical
medicine at Oxford, is one of Britain's leading clinical scientists;
Lewis Thomas, professor of paediatrics, pathology, medicine and
biology and dean of two medical schools, enjoys a similar status in
the USA. The discreet scepticism of these two eminent medical
authorities regarding the central themes of government public
health policy on both sides of the Atlantic indicates two things: that
some medical experts question the scientific basis of this policy –

and that this questioning has had done little to deter the rise of public health promotion to become a major influence in modern society and in the everyday lives of its citizens.

The 'big four' injunctions of health promotion – to stop smoking cigarettes, to eat a healthy diet, to drink alcohol in moderation, and take regular exercise – have become firmly established in popular consciousness. People may not heed the advice coming at them from the government, the media, the medical profession, but nobody can now be unaware of the key components of what is officially regarded as a healthy life. The huddles of furtive smokers outside ordinary houses as well as public buildings symbolise the ascendancy of preoccupations about health over social behaviour.

Over the past decade the reach of health promotion has widened and deepened. Each of the big four has expanded and become more differentiated. The evils of smoking have been compounded by the perils of passive smoking. Every schoolchild knows how to calculate the units of alcohol in different beverages and the approved limits for men and women. The merits of fruit and fibre and the dangers of saturated fatty acids have been ventilated in every kitchen in the nation, just as almost every household has an exercise bike and an aerobic workout video (however rarely used). Everybody is also now aware of the dangers of exposure to sunlight, how to put a baby to sleep to reduce the risk of cot death and of the requirements of safe sex. Medical jurisdiction over lifestyle now extends into the home, the workplace, the school and the neighbourhood. It also covers every moment of the life-cycle, from pre-conception counselling, through pregnancy and childbirth, infancy, childhood and adolescence, not merely women's health but also men's health, the menopause (and the male mid-life crisis), old age and death.

In this chapter we look at the evolution of some of the key themes in the regulation of lifestyle in the cause of health. The origins of current health promotion policies lie in the responses of modern medicine to the challenges of coronary heart disease and cancer, conditions whose importance increased dramatically in the mid-twentieth century as the menace of infectious disease receded. The demonstration, in the early 1950s, of the link between cigarette smoking and lung cancer was the towering achievement of modern epidemiology, providing the rationale for a strategy of prevention which has been fervently sought in relation to other diseases. Unfortunately, though numerous risk factors have been identified, no distinct causal agent has been discovered for any other common form of cancer or for heart disease. As a result, preventive strategies have had to fall back on attempts either to modify risk factors or to detect disease at an early stage.

The assumptions that prevention is better than cure and that early diagnosis is preferable to late diagnosis have a ready appeal – for both doctors and patients. This guarantees widespread popularity for health promotion policies, especially when the condition in question is a common cause of death and disability. Yet these assumptions may not be correct. Both health promotion policies and screening programmes involve interventions in the lives of the mass of the well in the hope of preventing diseases among a few. These interventions may cause considerable adverse consequences for some of the well, while not even benefiting many of the few, some of whom still succumb to the disease.

Yet, though all forms of health promotion have provoked medical and scientific controversy over their claims to effectiveness, they have steadily gained in public prestige and impact over the past two decades. As a result, interventions which originated in the world of medicine have long since acquired a wider social and political significance, so that they can no longer be understood exclusively, or even primarily, in medical terms. In the following chapters, we will be looking at screening programmes and at the political controversies around health promotion; here we focus on the 'big four' lifestyle issues targeted by health promotion activists.

Smoking

Deaths from lung cancer in Britain increased from around 300 a year in the early 1920s to more than 3,000 a year 20 years later. By the early 1960s the annual death rate reached 30,000, since when there has been a slow decline. Given the popularity of smoking – at its peak just after the Second World War, some 65 per cent of men in Britain smoked – it is not surprising that the discovery of the link between cigarettes and lung cancer has had a major impact on public life and personal behaviour. The controversy over smoking went through three phases up to the 1980s (a fourth, following the discovery of nicotine addiction, we examine in Chapter 6).

In the first phase, in the 1950s, the debate about tobacco was largely confined to the medical profession. In a series of classic papers, epidemiologist Richard Doll and statistician Austin Bradford Hill established the link between smoking and lung cancer, most convincingly in a major study of British doctors (RCP 1962).

The proportion of doctors who smoked fell from nearly 40 per cent in 1951 to just above 20 per cent ten years later (RCP 1962: 11). In the second phase, during the 1960s and 1970s, the campaign against smoking went public. This phase opened with the publication in Britain of the Royal College of Physicians' pamphlet *Smoking and Health*, and in the USA, with the Surgeon General's Report of the same title (RCP 1962; US Surgeon-General 1964). The 1964 ban on cigarette advertising on television was the first significant official restriction on the tobacco industry. In the early 1960s the proportion of adult male smokers declined from about 60 per cent to reach a level of around 52–53 per cent, where it stuck until the early 1970s. The proportion of women smokers remained fairly steady just above 40 per cent as did the tendency of manual workers to smoke more than professionals. The second edition of the RCP report in 1971 further implicated smoking in other forms of malignancy, respiratory and heart diseases, and complications of pregnancy (RCP 1971). It called for further restrictions on the advertising and sale of cigarettes (including warning notices on packets) and for bans on smoking in public places. This report prompted the formation of the campaigning group Action on Smoking and Health (ASH) which gave the anti-smoking cause a higher media profile. Smoking levels fell steadily from the early 1970s, among men and women, to reach a plateau at around 28 per cent in the mid-1990s.

The discovery of the dangers of 'passive smoking' in the 1980s marked the third phase of the tobacco wars and a decisive shift in the anti-smoking campaign. The first indication of this problem came in a paper from Japan in 1981; by 1986 the US Surgeon-General noted that some thirteen studies from five different countries had confirmed an increased risk (US Surgeon-General 1986). The resulting 1987 ban on smoking on US domestic air flights and the attendant controversy put the passive smoking issue decisively on the public agenda. In 1988, the Froggat Committee, an independent scientific committee on smoking and health, estimated that passive smoking caused an increased risk of lung cancer of between 10 and 30 per cent and recommended restrictions on smoking in workplaces and in public (Jackson 1995). The case against passive smoking gathered momentum through the 1990s. In 1992 the US Environmental Protection Agency declared 'environmental tobacco smoke' (ETS) a carcinogen, or cancer-causing agent (US EPA 1992). In 1997 the California Environmental Protection Agency added low birth weight babies, cot death, childhood asthma and nasal sinus cancer to the list of conditions caused by ETS (California EPA 1997). British meta-analyses confirmed increased risks of lung cancer (24 per cent) and coronary heart disease (23 per cent) (Hackshaw *et al.* 1997, Law *et al.* 1997). A re-analysis of the same studies three years later acknowledged a 'modest degree of publication bias' (a result of the fact that studies which reveal no increased risk are less likely to be published) and adjusted the excess risk of lung cancer down from 24 per cent to 15 per cent (Copas, Shi 2000)

The case against ETS transformed smoking from a self-endangering choice into an anti-social act. The smoker was not only engaging in a personally destructive practice, but one which was polluting the immediate environment and threatening a cast of 'innocent victims' – non-smoking spouses (generally wives), children, unborn babies. Parental smoking came to be regarded as little better than child abuse (indeed it soon became a significant barrier to adoption). The campaign led to the establishment of 'smoke-free' areas and then smoking bans in workplaces, on public transport and other public spaces. The award, by Stockport council in 1993, of £15,000 in damages to Veronica Bland, who claimed that her chronic bronchitis resulted from eleven years of exposure to smoking workmates, marked the public affirmation of the status of the passive smoker in Britain. As the medical historian Allan Brandt observed, 'in less than a decade, American public space was radically subdivided on the basis of the harms of passive smoking' (Brandt 1998).

Despite the growing medical (and political) consensus about the dangers of passive smoking, the issue has remained controversial. The Swedish toxicologist Robert Nilsson, while accepting the plausibility of the ETS-lung cancer link and the fact that numerous studies appear to show a statistically significant increase in risk, has questioned its epidemiological significance (Nilsson 1997). Thus he offered estimates, on the basis of current knowledge, of the annual incidence of cancer in a population of 100,000 resulting from various environmental factors: unknown (177), diet (135), smoking (68), other lifestyle factors (45), sunshine (23), ...ETS (2). By contrast, in a population which consumes Japanese seafood (which contains arsenic) this will cause 12 cases of cancer; where there are traces of natural arsenic in drinking water, this will cause five cases; eating mushrooms will cause three cases. In other words, the risk of ETS is comparable with that of environmental agents which are generally regarded as an insignificant threat to health.

Nilsson further questioned the biological plausibility of ETS as a risk factor. Even if the more moderate increases are true – and given that passive smoking has been estimated to be equivalent to actively smoking up to half a cigarette a day – the cancer-causing potency of ETS appears to be around ten times greater than mainstream smoke. Another anomaly of passive smoking is that it appears to be associated with an increased risk of a type of lung cancer that arises from glandular tissue (adenocarcinoma) instead of from the cells lining the airways (squamous or oat cell carcinoma) which is the familiar type caused by smoking. This type of tumour appears to be more common in East Asia – where many of the studies of passive smoking have been conducted. The idea that a very low level of smoke inhalation could cause a type of lung cancer in passive smokers that vastly higher levels do not appear to cause in heavy smokers defies biology and common sense. Nilsson also pointed to a number of possible sources of bias or confounding in the conduct and interpretation of studies of passive smoking. He also noted that the increased risk suggested by some surveys implies that passive smoking is more dangerous than smoking up to ten cigarettes a day.

Perhaps the most fundamental defect of the presentation of the risk of passive smoking is the failure to distinguish between relative and absolute risk. In a critical commentary, the Australian medical research scientist Raymond Johnstone noted that the annual death rate from lung cancer among the non-smoking wives of non-smoking men is around six per 100,000, whereas among the non-smoking wives of smoking men the corresponding figure is eight per 100,000. Now this may be reported as an increased (relative) risk of 33 per cent. Yet in absolute terms it amounts to an absolute (or exposure) risk of one in 50,000, which is, for practical purposes, negligible. His conclusion was that 'the most that one can say about the alleged link beween passive smoking and lung cancer is that if there is one, then it is so small that it is difficult to measure it accurately and the risk, if any, is well below the level of those to which we normally pay attention' (Johnstone 1991: 81). The alarming estimates of deaths attributable to passive smoking result from multiplying minuscule risks of dubious validity by vast population numbers – an effective propaganda device but statistical sharp practice.

The drive to impose restrictions on smoking in workplaces and in public has not been in the least inhibited by expert doubts about the validity of the evidence on which it is based. Indeed, as medical historian Virginia Berridge has observed, 'the coalition advocating those restrictions pre-dated the evidence' (Berridge 1998). Yet, as she acknowledged, 'by the mid-1990s, there was widespread agreement that the epidemiological evidence on passive smoking was at least debatable'. It may have been regarded as debatable among medical experts at an elite symposium, but as far as public policy was concerned ETS was lethal. In a revealing exchange at the same symposium on the history of smoking and health, when Richard Doll was asked to compare the epidemiological evidence on passive smoking with his work in the 1950s, his response was 'it's utterly different' (Doll 1998). Recalling that his study had shown a fifty-fold increase in risk for heavy smokers, he commented that 'for passive smoking the evidence is qualitatively different'. While indicating that he did believe that passive smoking was harmful, he conceded that 'the quantitative relationship is very weak', suggesting that his belief was more grounded in loyalty to the anti-smoking cause than his confidence in the figures.

Heart attack on a plate?

The discovery of the link between smoking and lung cancer gave a great impetus to the quest for some similar causative agent of coronary heart disease (CHD), another condition which caused a rapidly increasing death toll from the 1920s onwards. Mortality from coronary heart disease grew at an even faster rate, reaching twice the rate of lung cancer in the early 1950s and three times the rate in the 1960s. Sudden death from a heart attack, particularly affecting men in middle age – a condition virtually unknown before the First World War – became familiar throughout the Western world. The coronary death rate in Britain reached a plateau in the late 1970s and then slowly declined (in the USA, this fall began a decade earlier).

The cause of the rapid increase in CHD was (and largely re-mains) a mystery, as does the reason for its more recent decline (which began before any of the familiar preventive interventions had been implemented on a large scale). In the 1950s, studies of differences in coronary death rates in different countries led to the recognition of an association between diets high in saturated fats (in meat and dairy products) and heart disease. The factor linking dietary fat and the formation of fatty plaques on the lining of the coronary arteries, which in turn lead to the formation of blood clots causing heart attacks, appeared to be the level of cholesterol circulating in the blood stream. The resulting thesis that a diet low in fat could prevent or reverse these pathological processes and reduce the rates of resulting death and disease has subsequently become the conventional wisdom of Western society. The popular description of the traditional British fried breakfast as a 'heart attack on a plate' reflects the familiarity of the diet–heart disease thesis.

It is indeed a plausible theory, yet, despite decades of intensive study, it still lacks scientific verification. Through the 1960s and 1970s controversy raged over the significance of dietary fat and the association between cholesterol and CHD and numerous researchers studied different aspects of the alleged link. A major joint US/European study – the Multiple Risk Factor Intervention Trial (MR FIT) – investigated the effect of various diets and lifestyle changes on 60,000 men. Other investigators identified additional risk factors for coronary heart disease, notably smoking, lack of exercise, raised blood pressure, and many more.

At the end of 1982, according to James LeFanu, a long-standing critic of the cholesterol-heart disease thesis, 'the juggernaut crashed' (LeFanu 1999: 335). The MR FIT trial showed no benefit from intervention (and a WHO study a few months later came to the same conclusion). Furthermore, figures showed that the incidence of CHD was falling in different countries, in all ages, classes and ethnic minorities – apparently independently of dietary changes. Yet far from bringing to an end attempts to change diet justified by the cholesterol-heart disease thesis, campaigns promoting 'healthy eating' won ever greater official backing and became steadily more influential. This is the remarkable paradox underlying health promotion in relation to CHD, to which we will return in the next chapter. Here, we simply note the fundamental improbability of the diet–CHD thesis: human beings have lived throughout history, and continue to live, in the most diverse habitats on the most diverse diets, displaying phenomenal adaptability. It would therefore seem 'improbable that for some reason right at the end of the twentieth century subtle changes in the pattern of food consumption should cause lethal diseases' (LeFanu 1999: 319–20).

There can be no doubt however that, even though – in scientific terms – the cholesterol juggernaut had crashed, in the sphere of public health policy, it was surging ahead. In 1979 the British government published guidelines on *Eating for Health* which attempted to overcome the 'ignorance and irresponsibility' which it blamed for unhealthy lifestyle. The media responded to this initiative with 'unbounded enthusiasm', publicising the dangers of cholesterol to a receptive audience (Karpf 1988). The 'Look After Yourself' campaign was launched by the Health Education Council in 1977 and developed in the early 1980s in collaboration with the BBC through a series of popular radio and television programmes. This campaign took the healthy eating message to the people, providing special training for nurses and health visitors to run groups in GPs surgeries, community centres and workplaces. In the USA, the National Cholesterol Education Campaign was launched along similar lines in 1984.

The cholesterol controversy raged on into the 1990s. In 1992 a major trial on the prevention of CHD by reducing cholesterol levels and other risk factors revealed an *increase* in mortality among those who received medical intervention (Dunnigan 1993). Another report indicated an increase in non-cardiac deaths related to drug treatment for increased cholesterol levels. Two years later the pro-dietary intervention camp produced new epidemiological data confirming the association between circulating cholesterol levels and death from heart disease. It claimed 'conclusive' evidence from a number of large studies that a 10 per cent reduction in blood cholesterol level (over a five-year period) could produce a 25 per cent drop in heart attacks (or other coronary incidents) (Marmot 1994). Researchers also dismissed reports of the dangers of low cholesterol levels and the risks of cholesterol-lowering drugs (Law *et al.* 1994a).

In the *Health of the Nation* campaign launched by a White Paper in 1992, the government, the medical profession and the media combined forces to promote a healthy diet – defined above all as one low in saturated fats (DoH 1992). It set specific targets:

- to reduce the average percentage of food energy derived by the population from saturated fatty acids by at least 35 per cent by 2005
- to reduce the average percentage of food energy derived by the population from total fat by at least 12 per cent by 2005

Recognising that abstract targets and general exhortations would have little effect, the government produced numerous booklets and leaflets providing detailed practical advice and tips about healthy eating. The Health Education Authority promoted the same message through the media and through local campaigns. Reports from the top level government Cardiovascular Review Group

Committee on Medical Aspects of Food Policy offered further recommendations to the public on matters such as the number of portions of fruit and vegetables that should be eaten daily ('at least five') (COMA 1994).

Doctors were given professional responsibility for relaying the message of CHD prevention to members of the public at their most vulnerable – as patients. The new contract imposed on GPs in 1990 provided substantial cash incentives for health promotion, and the government particularly encouraged CHD prevention initiatives. Everybody was now entitled to a 'health check' on registering with a doctor: an interrogation about lifestyle and an examination featuring measurement of height, weight and blood pressure naturally culminated in a lecture on healthy eating and other aspects of a medically-approved lifestyle. Following the victory of New Labour in 1997, its public health policy documents restated the cholesterol–CHD link, but placed it in a wider lifestyle context. The government emphasised the importance of working through local initiatives in schools, workplaces and communities, in particular through health action zones and healthy living centres (DoH 1998, 1999). Though acknowledging the contribution of poverty to a poor diet and difficulties of access to affordable food, the White Paper emphasised that 'major changes in diet, particularly among the worst off, with increased consumption of such foods as fruit, vegetables and oily fish' would greatly reduce the risk of CHD (DoH 1999: 78)

Though it remains popular with the government, the medical profession and the public, the diet–CHD thesis is deeply flawed both as an explanation and as a preventive strategy. The association between cholesterol and CHD may be strong, but it is clearly not the only factor involved (Bonneux, Barendregt 1994). The incidence of CHD has been declining over many years in different Western populations, despite steady or even increasing levels of cholesterol. A major British study has shown that, though cholesterol levels tend to be lower in lower social classes, the incidence of CHD is around four times higher (Rose, Marmot 1981). Genetic, cultural and environmental factors, as well as chance, also appear to affect any particular individual's likelihood of acquiring CHD. This means that the scope for personal initiative in improving survival prospects is relatively small.

Advocates of the diet–CHD thesis tend to assume that the recommended reduction in blood cholesterol is easily achieved by dietary changes. According to one group of experts, this is not the case (Ramsey *et al.* 1994). Simple fat-reducing diets of the sort recommended by the familiar 'healthy eating' leaflets ('step 1') are well tolerated, but produce only marginal reductions in blood cholesterol levels. More drastic diets, which are required to achieve the target cholesterol reduction ('step 3') are widely regarded as unpalatable and cannot be sustained by most people. These authors recommended that proponents of the cholesterol thesis 'should apply the same rigour to assessing the effectiveness of intervention as they have to their analyses of the epidemiological and clinical trial data'.

Another limitation on the preventive value of dietary intervention is the fact that CHD is overwhelmingly a disease of the elderly – 83 per cent of people who die from CHD are over 65. The significance of this may be clarified by calculating the increase in life expectancy resulting from a fall in CHD mortality of 25 per cent (the consequence of a 10 per cent reduction in blood cholesterol levels): between 2.5 and 5.0 months (Bonneux and Barendregt 1994). In response to this (and another computer-modelled calculation which suggested the possibility of a median increase of 12 months), supporters of dietary intervention argued that the average increase over the whole population concealed the benefit to those who would otherwise die from CHD (for whom the increase was on average four years, and eight for those dying under fifty) (Law *et al.* 1994a). But this is a statistical sleight of hand: if dietary change is being recommended for everybody, then its benefit must be measured across the whole population. Faced with the choice between forgoing the pleasures of meat and cheese and prolonging a miserable fruit and fibre existence for a few more months, many people might opt to eat now and forfeit the few extra months.

The distinction between relative and absolute risk we considered in relation to passive smoking also applies to diet. It is important to distinguish between the apparently impressive improvement in the relative risk of CHD resulting from dietary change and the marginal improvement in absolute risk. Two American professors of medicine made this point in response to the 'cholesterol papers' debate in the BMJ in 1994:

> Most doctors answer in the affirmative when asked whether they would take a daily pill to reduce their chances of dying from a heart attack by 50 per cent. When asked whether they would do so for ten to twenty years if the risk

was reduced from 2/1000 to 1/1000, a reduction of 50 per cent, there is much less enthusiasm.

(Vine, Hastings 1994)

The chance of a forty-year-old man with a relatively high blood cholesterol dying from a heart attack are very small indeed. Reducing his cholesterol level by ten per cent would make his chances of such a death very, very small indeed. Such improvements, the authors concluded, 'may represent substantial epidemiological benefit' but are of 'trivial clinical importance'.

A man advised of his chances in these terms might well decide to live dangerously, but happily, on bacon and eggs, rather than marginally more safely on muesli and skimmed milk, with the added risk of dying miserable and flatulent.

The demon drink

There is no minimum threshold below which alcohol can be consumed without any risk ... Alcohol can be blamed for some of the world's most serious health problems ... We should be aware that alcohol is a risky, addictive and toxic substance.

(quoted in Craft 1994)

Every adult should have an alcohol consumption history taken using units of alcohol.

(Health of the Nation, An information pack for General Practitioners, 1992)

Patient: Will I live longer if I give up alcohol and sex?
Doctor: No, but it will seem like it.

(Cleare and Wessely 1997)

It is not immediately obvious why alcohol should have assumed such a high profile in the health promotion campaigns of recent years. Whereas smoking and cholesterol were both linked to diseases which had increased dramatically in prevalance, there was no such rise in conditions associated with alcohol. It has long been recognised, by the public as well as doctors, that acute intoxication sometimes induces violent or self-destructive behaviour and that chronic excess consumption leads to cirrhosis of the liver. In the past, public concerns about the damaging consequences of alcohol excess for the individual and society were expressed in the temperance movement. Closely aligned with evangelical Christianity, temperance campaigners regarded drunkenness as a moral failure and presented abstinence as the route to personal redemption. The anti-alcohol initiatives of the past decade have revived the puritanical spirit of the temperance movement, but in a modern, medicalised, form. Alcohol dependency is now regarded as a disease, though one affecting a growing proportion of the population.

Whereas the old temperance movement was dedicated to rescuing the 'habitual drunk', the medical temperance movement shifted the focus of attention, first from the 'alcoholic' to the 'problem drinker', and then to the whole of society. The key to this transition was the adoption of the system of calculating alcohol consumption by units. In 1979 the Royal College of Psychiatrists first indicated that a weekly consumption of more than 56 units of alcohol was the 'absolute upper limit'. In 1984 the Health Education Council suggested that weekly levels of between 21 and 36 units for men, and 14 and 24 units for women, would be 'unlikely to cause damage'. Then in the late 1980s a new consensus emerged from the royal colleges and other medical bodies, setting the upper limits at 21 for men and 14 for women that have been the basis of most subsequent guidelines (RCPsych 1986; RCGP 1988; RCP 1987; Medical Council on Alcoholism 1987).

Three things are worth noting about the process of quantifying alcohol consumption. The first is its arbitrary character: there is no strong scientific evidence for any of these figures, which are simply based on extrapolating from studies relating levels of alcohol consumption to manifestations of disease among heavy drinkers to the rest of society. The second is the trend for the limits to become tighter, a trend more related to the increasing sobriety of the wider political climate than to the emergence of epidemiological evidence justifying a more abstemious policy. The third is that, according to the 21/14 criteria, more than a quarter of men and more than one in ten women in Britain are drinking excessively. The medicalisation of alcohol has, in short, resulted in a dramatic inflation of the scale of the problem, justifying a more systematic intervention in the drinking habits of society.

In the *Health of the Nation* campaign in the early 1990s, the government set specific targets to reduce alcohol consumption. The White Paper noted research revealing that 28 per cent of men were drinking more than 21 units a week and 11 per cent of women were drinking more than 14 units a week. It then proposed to reduce the proportion of excessive male drinkers to 18 per cent and that of female drinkers to 7 per cent (by 2005) (DoH 1992). It was the specific task of GPs to 'advise patients to restrict their drinking to within the recommended daily levels for men and women' and to 'advise patients to avoid intoxication in inappropriate circumstances, e.g. drinking and driving, drinking in the workplace'.

The government's method of tackling the problems arising from the excessive consumption of alcohol by a small proportion of the population by attempting to restrict the alcohol consumption of the whole of society was an application of the 'population strategy' advocated by the epidemiologist Geoffrey Rose (Rose 1985). Rose's strategy was based on the recognition that the pattern of drinking in society, like that of other behaviours likely to cause a threat to health, was unevenly distributed, with relatively small numbers at either extreme and the bulk of the population falling in the moderate middle ground. Instead of following the traditional approach of concentrating on a few heavy drinkers, the population strategy set about shifting the whole pattern of drinking in society in a more moderate direction. The idea was that if everybody was drinking slightly less, then there would be fewer problem drinkers. The fallacy of this argument is readily apparent: it is quite possible for many moderate drinkers to reduce their drinking to an even more moderate level, while a few hard drinkers carry on just as before or even increase their intake (Charlton 1995, Swales 1995). The appeal of the population strategy to government is that it legitimises intervention in the personal behaviour of everybody, while avoiding the stigmatising character of any approach targeted specifically at problem drinkers.

Though the medical temperance campaign was eagerly taken up by health promotionists and radical epidemiologists, in the course of the 1990s it encountered some epidemiological difficulties of its own. In face of earlier research revealing the adverse effects of alcohol, not only on the liver, but in increasing risks of heart disease and cancer, new studies claimed to show that moderate drinking had a beneficial effect on health and longevity (Marmot, Brunner 1991). In particular a study conducted by a team headed by Richard Doll, famed for revealing the smoking–lung cancer link forty years earlier, concluded that 'among British men in middle or older age, the consumption of an average of one or two units of alcohol a day is associated with significantly lower all-cause mortality than is consumption of no alcohol, or the consumption of substantial amounts of alcohol' (Doll *et al.* 1994). It appeared that drinking a couple of glasses of wine a day had a 'cardio-protective' effect, reducing the risk of coronary heart disease. Doll's paper provoked an angry denunciation from the director of the World Health Organisation's 'programme on substance abuse', whose response is quoted at the head of this section. The WHO was concerned that the publicity given to this study might encourage people to start drinking: 'we are seeking to demystify the idea that alcohol is good for your health and to debunk the idea that to have a drink a day will keep the doctor away' (Craft 1994).

The following year, the royal colleges reviewed their anti-alcohol guidelines in the light of the discovery that the graph of mortality against alcohol intake was not linear, but 'J-shaped'. These eminent medical authorities acknowledged the new research but recommended that there should be no change from the current 21/14 recommendations, which were 'prudent' and 'justified' (indeed Doll *et al.* had not suggested any change) (RCP, RCPsych, RCGP 1995). However, in December 1995, in an apparent surge of Christmas cheer, the government announced new guidelines, recommending limits of 3–4 units a day for men and 2–3 units a day for women (DoH 1995). Though health minister Stephen Dorrell denied any intention of raising the threshold of 'sensible drinking', simple arithmetic revealed new weekly limits of 28 for men and 21 for women. This statement was immediately branded a 'boozers' charter' in the tabloid press and as fervently condemned by the anti-alcohol movement as it was welcomed by the drink trade. The BMA described the government's initiative as 'both irresponsible and badly timed' and the Royal College of Physicians complained that 'by raising the "sensible limits" people are being encouraged to drink more' (*Times*, 13 December 1995).

The controversy over the dangers and benefits of alcohol rumbled on. This is how two leading epidemiologists posed the problem confronting health promotionists in this area:

> Is it possible to persuade older non-drinkers to drink a little for the benefit of their health, and is it possible to do this without increasing the number of people, especially teenagers, who drink at levels that are dangerous?
>
> (White, McKie 1997)

This comment confirms both the remoteness of health promotionists from the real world and the absurdity of the debate about alcohol and health. For the vast majority of people, whether they are teetotallers or drunks, or at some point on the wide spectrum in between, concerns about health are not a significant factor in their drinking behaviour. People may drink alcohol in varying quantities (or may not drink at all) for all sorts of cultural, social and psychological reasons. In my experience most habitual heavy drinkers are well aware that alcohol does not have a beneficial effect on their health, but reminding them of this does not inhibit their consumption. People who drink only occasionally or not at all have their own reasons, among which concerns about health are not likely to be prominent. Only an epidemiologist could believe that either a middle aged non-drinker sitting at home or a teenager going out on a weekend is going to be influenced by government propaganda advising them of the health benefits of 'sensible drinking'. But then only an epidemiologist could believe that data based on 'self-reported' levels of alcohol consumption can provide a useful basis for quantitative studies.

The power of the ideology of health promotion is such that even its critics sometimes fall back on attempts to justify a particular lifestyle choice in terms of health. Thus, campaigners against the tyranny of counting units of alcohol in different beverages have seized on associations between moderate levels of alcohol consumption and reduced mortality to bolster their case. As Dalrymple observes, 'even those who warn against health fanatics forget their own principles when an association emerges that pleases them' (Dalrymple 1998). Both arguments, based – like most of the epidemiology underlying health promotion – on the confusion of association with causation, are equally irrational. Opponents of the 'health fanatics' would be on stronger ground if they pointed out that drinking alcohol in its wonderful diversity of forms is a highly pleasurable activity which has, in general, nothing to do with health. The familiar fact that some people drink an excessive amount of alcohol, causing adverse physical, psychological and social consequences, is strictly irrelevant to the drive to regulate the drinking habits of the entire population in the name of health.

Exercise

Over the past couple of years I have been able to refer my patients to an 'Exercise on Prescription' scheme organised by Hackney Council 'education and leisure' services in collaboration with the local health authority (Hackney Education and Leisure 1997).

Under this scheme I can refer patients to a local leisure centre for a twelve week exercise programme, beginning with 'a thirty minute consultation with the health and fitness adviser'. They will then 'be asked to attend at least two sessions a week' of activities, including 'low intensity keep fit sessions', 'aqua-aerobics and learn-to-swim sessions', a 'walking programme', 'personal fitness programmes' and 'cardiac rehabilitation programmes'. Though the scheme is subsidised, participants are asked to pay between £1 and £2 per session. By 1999 more than 200 such schemes were in operation around the country and were reportedly popular with patients, doctors (and with leisure centres which gained a steady supply of customers during times of low demand).

It may seem perverse to criticise a campaign to encourage people to take more exercise, something that many would regard as self-evidently beneficial. Yet it is important to note the subtly coercive character of these exercise programmes. As a doctor, I do not advise or recommend exercise, but I prescribe it, in the same manner as I would a drug or other medical treatment. As the programme leaflet indicates, 'an exercise prescription is similar to a prescription for medicine issued by your GP ... in many cases exercise can help to control certain medical conditions and in some cases reduce the need for medication'. The deliberate use of the term 'prescription' implies an expectation that the patient will follow the doctor's instructions to turn up at the gym, just as they would be expected to take a traditional prescription to the pharmacy and take the medication in the manner prescribed: 'all patients should be made aware of the fact that the prescription is an important part of their treatment'. Issuing a prescripton to take exercise clearly imposes a much greater pressure for compliance on the patient than there would be if the doctor merely advised exercise.

Doctors were not always such enthusiasts for physical exertion. In the past, they have often warned of the dangers of particular sports and have complained about the burden on accident and emergency and orthopaedic departments resulting from sports injuries. In 1990 the BMA published a detailed account of the dangers of sporting and leisure activities, noting 155 fatalities in 1987, including some 61 drownings in various water sports, 24 deaths from parachuting, hang-gliding and other forms of aerial recreation, 12 from horse-riding and jumping (though only one in boxing, the target of a continuing medical campaign) (BMA 1990: 147–8). According to one estimate, around 1.5 million injuries caused by exercise are seen by doctors every year, resulting in the loss of 5.5 million working days (Nicholl 1992). The growing popularity of more dangerous sports, like mountain climbing and off-piste skiing, has led to an increase in sport-related mortality, despite the increasing preoccupation with safety.

Two factors have converged to make exercise a key feature of the modern health promotion agenda. One is the burgeoning cult of the body that has become a central theme of Western society over the past twenty years. This began with the vogue for jogging and marathon running in the 1970s and 1980s and has flourished in the form of gym-based fitness training in the 1990s. People seem to have forgotten that Pheidippides, the runner of the first marathon in 490 BC, collapsed and died on reaching Athens – and that James Fixx, who popularised jogging in the USA with his 1977 best-seller, dropped dead on the track in 1984 at the age of 52 (Skrabanek 1994: 74–5). The second factor is the increasing medical promotion of the preventive value of exercise in relation to a wide range of health problems, from coronary heart disease and osteoporosis, to depression and anxiety.

In 1991 the Royal College of Physicians reviewed the medical aspects of exercise, balanced the benefits and risks and pronounced that regular exercise conferred definite 'physical and psychosocial benefits' (RCP 1991). It recommended the promotion of exercise from childhood to old age and advised doctors to 'ask about exercise', while recognising the risks. In the *Health of the Nation* campaign launched the following year, exercise was a key theme. The campaign's information pack for GPs claimed that inactivity doubled the risk of CHD and tripled the risk of stroke, whilst exercise prevented osteoporosis and diabetes. One of 'the main messages' for GPs was to 'encourage people to be more active in daily living, and to aim for 30 minutes of moderate intensity activity (such as a brisk walk) on at least five days of the week'.

In the course of the subsequent debate about the *Health of the Nation* programme, two defenders of its emphasis on the promotion of exercise responded to their critics:

> 'Some would argue that there is no conclusive evidence from controlled trials that regular exercise reduces the number of deaths from coronary heart disease or substantially prolongs life. To demand such proof is to miss the point about exercise, which is that it is valuable for numer-

ous other health benefits it confers and as a catalyst in the adoption of a healthier lifestyle.

(Dargie, Grant 1992)

Given that a major national effort was being invested in promoting exercise on the grounds that it prevented heart disease, it seems fair enough to ask for evidence to substantiate this claim. Yet these exercise enthusiasts duck this demand, countering with an assurance that it confers numerous other health benefits. No doubt to ask for evidence of these benefits would also be to miss the point, which is that the health promoters firmly believe that exercise is conducive to a healthier lifestyle. It would appear to be faith rather than science that justifies medical calls to the public to take up exercise.

When the first 'exercise on prescription' schemes emerged in the early 1990s, medical commentators were sceptical. An editorial in the *BMJ* in 1994 recommended that 'primary health care teams should look closely before they leap into prescribing exercise. There may be many more effective ways for them to use their resources to increase the fitness of their practice populations' (Iliffe *et al.* 1994). Five years later a major randomised controlled trial of exercise on prescription in Newcastle found that 'short term increases in physical activity were not maintained at one year follow up and even the most intensive intervention was ineffective in promoting long-term adherence to increased physical activity' (Harland *et al.* 1999). Despite the conclusion from this study that health authorities should reconsider their investment of scarce resources in ineffective exercise on prescription schemes, they remain a prominent feature of the 'healthy living centres', the flagship project of New Labour's public health programme.

Our brief survey of lifestyle intervention in the cause of promoting better health reveals that the advice to stop (or not start) smoking is the one aspect of health promotion for which there is a rational basis. The problem is that people (often people who are poorer or more socially isolated) continue to smoke, not because they are unaware of the dangerous consequences for their health, but because, in the straitened circumstances of their lives, they derive considerable satisfaction from it. Research confirms that many regard smoking as a means of regulating mood and managing stress, as an activity which helps them to cope with the difficulties of everyday life (Graham 1987). Sociologist Hilary Graham, who went to the trouble of asking women why they smoked, found that women who were alone with young children reported that having a cigarette was 'the one thing they do for themselves', a moment of respite from the relentless work of caring (Graham 1994). In these circumstances, exhortations to stop smoking – or measures to increase the price of cigarettes – are not likely to have much effect. Yet as GPs we are constantly advised to seize the opportunity offered by patients' attendance at the surgery seeking medical advice or treatment for some different problem to inform them about the dangers of smoking and other lifestyle risk factors. Even when such advice is scientifically justified (which, as we have seen, it often is not) it is impertinent, especially if the recipient is ill. If the patient is a smoker and complains of a smoking related illness, the last thing they need is a doctor telling them what they already know about the evils of smoking and the virtues of a healthy lifestyle.

4

SCREENING

In 1971 Carol Downer stole a speculum from her doctor's office in Los Angeles and, aided by a mirror and a flashlight, became possibly the first woman in history to see her own cervix. Within twelve months she was running a women's self-help health group, turning to alternative medicine to treat vaginal discharges with such household remedies as yoghurt. The clinic was subsequently raided by the Los Angeles Police Department and she was charged with entering a vagina without a medical license. The LAPD attempted to seize as evidence a pot of yoghurt but were restrained by a woman who insisted it was her lunch. The incident quickly became known as the Great Yoghurt Bust and went on to make its appearance in court as the Great Yoghurt Trial. Downer was acquitted, thus establishing a precedent in California: women's genitals were no longer territory reserved for men.

(Linda Grant, *Sexing the Millennium*, 1993 p. 179)

Perhaps the last word on the subject [of cervical smears] can be left to a consultant pathologist, A.R. Kittermaster, writing in *World Medicine*. He felt diffident, he explained, about giving advice on screening for a disease which, as a man, he could not contract. When he considered a roughly equivalent disease which he might get, such as cancer of the prostate, he would certainly be willing to have the equivalent test if he had suspicious symptoms; 'but if anyone – and particularly a female – suggested that young men should start having regular smears to diagnose and treat pre-malignant lesions, twenty years before the average age for invasive cancer, I should be highly suspicious of the whole affair'. Certainly he would want proof that treatment in such circumstances had a dramatic effect on the death-rate;

and if he knew (as he did for cervical lesions) that having a smear carried an unavoidable risk of an incorrect diagnosis, 'then I would tell whoever was advocating the smear to go jump in the lake and poke their nose – or rather, their finger – somewhere else'.

(Brian Inglis, *The Diseases of Civilisation*, 1981 p. 69)

Within twenty years the feminist campaign to seize control over women's health from the medical profession had given way to state-sponsored, doctor-led systems of vaginal examination and cervical surveillance. It is doubly ironic that within the same period, male resistance to medical regulation was replaced by the demand, under the banner of 'men's health', for invasive screening tests analagous to cervical smears. Whereas the early women's movement rejected medical inspection of the cervix as an act of symbolic domination, the modern men's health movement invited rectal penetration as a symbol of its subordination to medical authority.

Given the failure of modern medicine to discover the causes of most forms of cancer, which might lead to a strategy of prevention, an obvious alternative was to devise some means of early detection, leading to prompt treatment and, hopefully, a better prognosis. For cancer of the cervix (neck of the womb) and the breast, screening tests have become popular over the past two decades, especially over the 1990s, when they were made available through national programmes and taken up by a large majority of the eligible population. These screening programmes claim substantial benefits in terms of reduced mortality – though in both cases these claims have been questioned by experts in the field. In recent years both programmes, but particularly the cervical smear scheme, have been subject to exposures of poor standards in some areas, leading to scares, scandals and litigation. As each screening test has specific features, let's take them in turn.

Smears

By offering screening to 250, 000, we have helped a few, harmed thousands, disappointed many, used £1.5m each year, and kept a few lawyers at work.

(Raffle 1997)

Cancer of the cervix is a fairly rare form of cancer in Britain, accounting for less than half a per cent of cancer deaths and around 4 per cent of cancer cases in women. Deaths from cervical cancer have slowly declined over the past 50 years, from 2,500 in 1950 to 1,150 in 1997 (Quinn *et al.* 1999). In 15 years as a GP I have had two patients who have died from cervical cancer, which is probably over the career average; typically, neither had ever had a smear test.

The smear test was introduced in Britain in the mid-1960s, following a famous study in British Columbia in Canada. This study appeared to show a dramatic reduction in cancer following the introduction of smear tests, which allowed the early detection and treatment of 'pre-cancerous' areas. There was considerable controversy at the time over whether the decline in death rate could be attributed to smear tests (it had declined elsewhere without such tests) and over whether cells labelled as 'pre-cancerous' might return to normal without treatment, rather than progressing to invasive malignancy. Smear tests failed to meet two of the standard criteria for screening programmes laid down by the World Health Organisation: cervical cancer is uncommon and its natural course is not well understood (Wilson, Jungner 1968). Though many experts were sceptical, a powerful lobby of cancer specialists prevailed upon the Labour government to introduce a cervical smear service in 1966 (Inglis 1981: 66–69).

Two years later the eminent epidemiologist Archie Cochrane caused a furore when he claimed that there was no evidence that smears would reduce the death rate from cervical cancer. He particularly objected to the use of a screening test for a condition for which there was no effective treatment (an authoritative review in 1999 conceded that there had been 'no significant improvements in treatment for cervical cancer over the past 20 years') (Quinn *et al.* 1999). Reflecting some years later on the 'uproar, abuse and isolation' he experienced as a result of his questioning of the cervical smear programme, Cochrane commented that, because of the introduction of this programme without proper evaluation, 'we would never know whether smears were effective or not' (Cochrane 1976: 260).

In 1988, following criticisms of the haphazard character of the cervical smear system, a National Coordinating Network for the NHS Cervical Screening Programme was established. In 1990 the new contract imposed on GPs by the government offered substantial incentives, now worth around £65 million a year, tied to smear rate performance targets. As a result of these measures, coverage of the target age group rose from 42 per cent in 1988 to 85 per cent in

1994, a level subsequently maintained (Quinn *et al.* 1999). The claim by these authors that in women under 55 'screening may have prevented 800 deaths in 1997' was contested by critics who noted that the data presented could equally well support the conclusion that screening caused a similar increase in mortality (Vaidya, Baum 1999).The contrast between the high level of public faith in the cervical smear programme and the private recognition among medical authorities of its unsatisfactory character is remarkable. In their reply to Vaidya and Baum, Quinn and his colleagues admitted that they remained 'deeply concerned about the well known problems with cervical screening', which they listed:

> cervical cancer is a comparatively rare disease and its natural course is not well understood; the smear test has both low sensitivity and low specificity; many tests are technically unsatisfactory and the proportion of such tests varies across the country; the mix of three-year and five-year screening intervals is inequitable; too many smear tests are opportunistic; and the programme costs four times as much as breast screening.
>
> (Quinn *et al.* 1999)

The low sensitivity of the smear test means that every year women are diagnosed as having cervical cancer which had been missed on previous smears. The fact that some such cases have resulted in litigation has led to calls for doctors to make clear that smears may miss between 5 and 15 per cent of abnormalities and to ensure that patients are giving properly informed consent to this procedure (Anderson 1999; Nottingham 1999).

The low specificity of the smear test means that it yields a relatively high proportion of false positive results: that is, it suggests that a woman has malignant or pre-malignant cells when more invasive procedures (involving the removal of a wider area of tissue in a 'loop' or 'cone' biopsy) confirm that this is not the case. In day to day practice, this is by far the biggest problem arising from smear tests, causing enormous anxiety and distress, often continuing for weeks or months pending delays in further investigations. Bristol public health consultant Angela Raffle noted the tendency of staff, in response to publicity over missed cases, to over-diagnose minor abnormalities (Raffle *et al.* 1995). While patients suffered needless anxiety, staff lived in fear of failing to identify potentially malignant cases. As a result, 'much of our effort in Bristol is devoted to limiting the harm done to healthy women and to protecting our staff from litigation as cases of serious disease continue to occur'. As Raffle recognised, many healthy women are left with worries about cancer and difficulties in obtaining life insurance. Those who receive treatment may experience considerable discomfort, bleeding and sexual problems – as well as long-term anxieties about fertility. Meanwhile women in that 10 to 15 per cent of the female population which has never had a smear, who are likely to be (like my two patients), older, poorer and from ethnic minorities, will ensure that the mortality figures remain fairly steady. Health promotion propaganda which characterises cervical cancer as a sexually transmitted disease (on the dubious grounds of an association with the wart virus) has undoubtedly deterred many women from having smear tests.

The annual cost of the cervical cancer screening programme is £132 million (Quinn *et al.* 1999). This is about four times the cost of the breast screening programme – though the death rate from breast cancer is around ten times greater.

Mammography

Breast cancer is not only much more common than cancer of the cervix, but the number of cases has gradually increased over the past twenty years. After rising slowly through the 1970s and 1980s, the death rate declined in the 1990s. There are currently around 30,000 cases a year, accounting for one-third of cancer in women; breast cancer kills around 11,000 women every year, causing around one-fifth of female cancer deaths. In our surgery we see several new cases of breast cancer every year and one or two deaths. We see many more women who turn out not have breast cancer but are understandably terrified by the appearance of a lump or other breast symptoms.

Trials of mammography – X-ray examination of the breast – for early detection of malignancy were carried out in the USA in the 1960s. Early results showed a resulting reduction in mortality among women over the age of fifty, but no benefit in younger women (Wells 1998). More extensive research in the 1970s confirmed the earlier results and mammography became established as a screening test for breast cancer. In Britain a national screening programme became operational in 1988; now women between the ages of 50 and 64 are invited for free mammography every three years. The combination of mammography with ultrasound and the microscopic study of cells extracted from a suspicious lump through 'fine needle aspiration' has greatly improved the diagnostic sensitivity of this process in the 1990s.

In 1995 the organisers published the results of the first five years of the mammography programme and claimed some credit for an 11 per cent drop in mortality from breast cancer in the target age group (Beral *et al.* 1995). In response, Professor Michael Baum, who had helped to set up the screening service, pointed out that though the mammography programme could not be expected to have an effect on mortality before 1997, the decline in the death rate began in 1985. Suggesting that a more likely explanation was the introduction of the drug Tamoxifen for the treatment of breast cancer, he argued that 'to claim that any part of this 11 per cent fall is attributable to the screening programme is intellectually dishonest' (Baum 1995). In protest, he resigned from the Department of Health's breast cancer screening advisory group.

Baum also pointed to the high level of false positive results generated by mammography, causing anxiety and leading to further investigations, either aspiration cytology or excision biopsy. He concluded that mammography was 'not worth doing' because it saved too few lives at too high a cost, while causing needless anxiety among thousands of healthy women by incorrectly suggesting that they have the disease (Rogers 1995). He suggested that the money spent on screening might be better spent on research and specialist treatment for women diagnosed with breast cancer. But breast cancer screening had acquired high political prestige; only three months earlier a parliamentary select committee had commended the mammography programme as a model of excellence in preventive health care and had called for it to be extended to cover women up to the age of 69. Baum's proposals were ignored.

The controversy over breast screening flared up again five years later. A study by a team from Denmark reviewed major trials of mammography in Sweden, Scotland, Canada and the USA, involving 500,000 women, and concluded that there was 'no reliable evidence that screening decreases breast cancer mortality' (Gotzsche, Olsen 2000). Prominent representatives of the government screening programme and the leading cancer charities immediately rejected this conclusion and asserted their conviction that mammography saved lives. Delyth Morgan, chief executive of Breakthrough Breast Cancer, insisted that 'we must not be deterred from continuing our screening programmes until we have seen categorically that they are ineffective' (*Guardian*, 7 January 2000).

This ethical imperative to prove a negative stood in dramatic contrast to the one imposed twenty years earlier in what has become recognised as a classic paper (Cochrane, Holland 1971). These authors distinguished between 'everyday medical practice', in which a patient asks for help and the doctor 'does the best he can', and the 'very different position' when the doctor 'initiates screening procedures'. In this situation, the doctor should 'have conclusive evidence that screening can alter the natural history of disease in a significant proportion of those screened'. By the turn of the millennium the science and ethics of screening were subordinated in the mammography programme to a combination of the government's need to maintain a high profile of concern for both health and women's issues, medical vested interests, the demands of the powerful cancer charities – and women's anxieties.

Public anxieties about breast cancer were encouraged by the official campaign to raise 'breast awareness'. October 1996 was designated Breast Cancer Awareness Month and, following the style set by the adoption of a red ribbon by Aids activists, a pink ribbon became a badge of breast awareness. Breast cancer won celebrity endorsements and became fashionable. One of the main effects of the promotion of breast cancer awareness is that it generates an exaggerated sense of risk. The Cancer Research Campaign promoted the estimate that '1 in 12' women will develop breast cancer, which featured on a nationwide poster campaign. According to an authoritative review, this was 'correct only for women who have escaped a number of equally serious but more likely threats to life at an earlier age' (Bunker *et al.* 1998). The authors concluded that 'for most women, the lifetime risk of dying of breast cancer is only 1 in 26; the other 25 will die of something else'.

Most of the women who come into the surgery worried about breast lumps are young, that is, under 50 – though the vast majority of deaths from breast cancer are in women over 65. Only one woman in 136 in Britain dies of breast cancer before the age of 50. Though the risk of dying from breast cancer increases with age, it appears to progress more slowly in older women, so that they often live long enough to die from some other cause. One of the ironies of discussing the risks of breast cancer is that, if the woman smokes, she has a greater risk of dying from lung cancer; even if she is a non-smoker, she is far more likely to die of heart disease. Public awareness of breast cancer has intensified the demand for screening tests which promise early diagnosis. The most basic is the technique of breast self-examination, which is generally recognised to be much more effective in generating anxiety than it is at detecting tumours (Austoker 1994a). Women's magazines and health promotion leaflets are still offering detailed diagrams and earnest advice about how to detect lumps – resulting in a steady flow of frightened women, some scarcely out of their teens, who are more likely to win the national lottery than to have breast cancer.

Another consequence of greater breast cancer awareness is the demand to extend mammography to women in their 40s. According to one commentator, this has provoked a debate in the USA 'out of proportion to its potential impact on public health' (Wells 1998). Despite the fact that numerous trials have failed to confirm the efficacy of this technique in younger women – and despite concerns that the radiation exposure involved might do greater harm – political pressures resulting from disease awareness campaigns have resulted in younger women having mammograms.

Women who have had breast cancer are perhaps the greatest casualties of breast awareness. It is not only that they are reminded of their disease every time they turn on the television or open a newspaper or magazine – and every time they see a pink ribbon on the bus or train. The popular discussion of the role of lifestyle factors in predisposing women to breast cancer compounds women's worries about their future with guilty reflections on their past behaviour. This is encouraged by epidemiological surveys which report the loosest of associations as causal influences. Thus the risk of breast cancer appears to be increased in women who have no children or who have them after the age of 30; in women who have taken the oral contraceptive pill or hormone replacement therapy; in women who drink alcohol and have a high fat diet. The relatively strong influence of family history on chances of getting breast cancer provides further scope for recriminations about genetic destiny and fatalistic ruminations about dying a premature and disfiguring death.

During breast awareness week, a patient of mine who has survived mastectomy, radiotherapy and chemotherapy and now has a good prognosis, came in to ask me what she had done to deserve breast cancer. I don't know who benefits from breast awareness, but I know many of its victims.

Carrying on screening

Despite all the problems of the cervical cytology and mammography programmes, the demand for more screening tests for other cancers continues to rise. One of the main sources of such demands in the late 1990s was the burgeoning men's health movement, associated with the wave of men's magazines, one of the publishing successes of the decade. Though it lacked the early radical impulse of feminism, the men's health movement adopted the later preoccupation of some feminists with health as their model. Far from challenging medical authority, men's health promoters urged men to submit themselves to it on a greater scale than ever before. In choosing campaigning issues, they proceeded by analogy with the feminists: they had cervical smears – we demand prostate examinations; they can do breast self-examination – we can feel our testicles. 'Perhaps', mused one urologist, 'there was a subliminal male desire to have a disease all of our own, even if it had to be a cancer' (Whelan 1997).

Though prostate cancer is relatively common in older men (95 per cent of 15,000 cases a year occur in men over 60), testicular cancer is a rare disease of younger men (causing around 100 deaths a year). Though treatment is often effective for both cancers, screening tests for early detection are generally considered unreliable. To detect prostate cancer it is possible to have a regular digital rectal examination, a blood test for the Prostate Specific Antigen, and a local ultrasound scan, but the predictive value of all these tests is low. Urologist Peter Whelan suggested that 'Promotes Stress and Anxiety' was an accurate description of the effect of the blood test. Given the rarity of testicular tumours, a high rate of false positive results is the inevitable outcome of any promotion of self-examination (Austoker 1994b).

It is however striking that, long after medical authorities have accepted the ineffectiveness of screening tests like the PSA, or self-examination of breasts and testicles, pressure groups and popular magazines continue to promote them. The extent of popular approval of these techniques, which is grossly disproportionate to any value they might have in reducing the impact of cancer, is a potent indicator of the pathological preoccupation with health that now prevails in society. It is ironic that young women are often advised to examine their breasts every month – an arbitrarily selected frequency that happens to coincide with the menstrual cycle – though the large majority of women with breast cancer are post-menopausal. Similarly, young men now turn up at the surgery after reading about prostate cancer in their men's magazines and request screening for a condition that only rarely appears before retirement age. The parallel between screening tests for cervical and prostatic cancer is symbolic. Just as the smear test exposes women not merely to the medical gaze but to vaginal penetration, so the palpation of the prostate involves digital penetration of the male rectum. The slippery finger may be less impressive than the metal speculum, but it is no less significant as an instrument of symbolic domination.

For its advocates screening has become an article of faith. Rejecting the evidence of the ineffectiveness of mammography, Delyth Morgan of Breakthrough Breast Cancer insisted that 'what we should be debating is how best to screen women' (*Guardian*, 7 January 2000). This response provides striking confirmation of the observation made fifteen years earlier in another critique of screening: 'In "keeping the faith", screening advocates may find themselves forced to accept or reject evidence not so much on the basis of its scientific merit as on the extent to which it supports or rejects the stand that screening is good' (Sackett, Holland 1975). The danger of this approach is not only that it leads to the continuation of costly and ineffective programmes. It also means that the harms of screening are passed over in silence: to mention them could discourage people from taking up the offer of testing. Indeed this was the first concern of the cancer charities in response to reports of the Danish study of mammography quoted above; public reassurances about the quality of the national cervical screening programme accompany every exposure of poor standards. Yet the harms resulting from screening are substantial: for every woman who benefits, tens of thousands undergo testing and hundreds receive unnecessary treatment. In presenting screening as an unequivocal benefit to women, doctors become advocates of state policy rather than of their patients' interests.

State intervention in personal life

In the screening programme the author was assigned an 'adviser' who would 'help her with her health' on an ongoing basis and monitor her progress towards 'better health'. The extensive questionnaire 'Taking the first step to better health' included the tendentious and extraordinarily patronising statement that the screening 'has been devised to help you change the way you look after your health. [It] is a programme of pro-active, preventive, care, dedicated to monitoring your health on an ongoing basis with the aim to give you a new, positive view on how to stay healthy in the years ahead'. The author took umbrage at (a) the assumption that she was not healthy already, and (b) the assumption she didn't know how to look after herself ...

The questionnaire also included a 'Women's section' of questions from the banal to the intrusively, impertinently and offensively intimate to 'help her with her health'. The author objected and was told that she was unusual in questioning the questions (most women, apparently don't because they trust doctors and have been brainwashed into believing that they need this nonsense). Suffice it to say, it was downhill after that.

(Ruth Lea, *Healthcare in the UK: The Need for Reform*, 2000 p. 77)

A number of themes emerge from our discussion of medical intervention in the cause of the prevention and early detection of disease. Over the past twenty years there has been, in the name of health promotion, a dramatic increase in state intervention in the personal life of the individual – ironically in a period when the state has been inclined to withdraw from economic and social commitments. The immediate consequence has been a stricter regulation of individual behaviour, though because this has been justified in the cause of improving the health of both the individual and the nation, it has not generally been experienced as coercive. The changed relationship between the state and the individual that is reflected in the greatly enhanced role of health has also changed the role of the medical profession and has given rise to a range of new institutions and professionals working in the sphere of health promotion.

The origins of each of the lifestyle interventions we have examined lie within the world of medicine and its attempts to tackle the 'modern epidemics' of heart disease and cancer. However, as is clear from our brief survey of the development of these interventions, at a certain point each was taken up by the state and transformed into a major national initiative. In the case of smoking, this occurred with the shift of focus to passive smoking in the late 1980s; in relation to CHD, government promotion of 'healthy eating' began earlier but also became a major campaign in the late 1980s and in the *Health of the Nation* initiatives of the early 1990s; both the cervical and breast screening programmes were nationalised in 1987–88.

The state's assumption of a leading role in health promotion inevitably changed the character of these initiatives. Once they had acquired a wider political and ideological role, their contribution to health became of secondary importance. At a time when politicians were preoccupied with the declining prestige of government, projecting an image of concern with health helped to shore up public approval. Successive governments recognised the potential of health as a means of establishing points of contact between the state and an increasingly atomised society, a trend which reached its apotheosis in NHS Direct, the 24-hour telephone advice line set up in 1999, claimed by Tony Blair as one of the greatest achievements of his first 1,000 days in office.

Employers too recognised the potential of health promotion in managing relations with workers. In a perceptive study, Margaret May and Edward Brunsdon noted the shift in the 1980s away from traditional 'occupational health' concerns towards 'new "wellness" interventions', including medical 'check-ups', 'health risk appraisal', screening tests and preventive lifestyle advice (May, Brunsdon 1994). They characterised this as 'a new form of employee control', far beyond the familiar organisation of work, as the jurisdiction of the employers extended into workers' private lives. They commented on the convergence of management theory and government health policy around the themes of personal responsibility. The proliferation of workplace smoking bans in the 1990s was another indication of the extension of managerial authority justified by concern for employee's welfare.

As health promotion assumed an ever greater profile, there was some divergence between the ways in which prevention strategies were presented to the public and how they were perceived within the private world of medicine. The politicians and the media wanted simple messages, soundbites, and doctors who took the lead in health promotion campaigns were happy to provide them – on the evils of passive smoking, the dangers of dairy products or the need for screening tests. Meanwhile, as we have seen, a high – and often increasing – level of scepticism came to prevail among medical experts about the value of all these interventions. In fact, in private, many doctors in all specialities are doubtful of the value of much of the work of health promotion. However, recognising the strength of the health promotion consensus, solidly backed by government funding, medical vested interests and compliant journalists, they think it best to keep their reservations to themselves. Indeed, as any of the sceptics who have spoken out could testify, the price of making private reservations about fashionable health promotion interventions public is high. The intellectual insecurity underlying the health promotion consensus is expressed in a dogmatic intolerance of criticism and intense hostility towards any dissident opinion. Anybody who ventures criticism of these policies – or has the temerity to publish research revealing their ineffectiveness – can expect a tirade of abuse and little prospect of academic advancement. A spirit of 'not in front of the children' governs debate as medical science is subordinated to political expediency.

The second theme that emerges from our discussion of health promotion interventions is the resulting restriction on individual liberty. This is not so much a matter of direct compulsion, but of the oppressive effect – well expressed by Bridget Jones in her eponymous diary – of living in constant awareness of the need to count cigarettes, calories and units of alcohol (Fielding 1997).

When I first received a 'health risk assessment' report resulting from the sort of encounter that so incensed Ruth Lea of the Institute of Directors in the account quoted above, I expected that it would provoke a similar response from many patients annoyed by the intrusive and impertinent character of the questions and the patronising style of the advice. In fact, such responses are strikingly uncommon. The attitude of most people to such procedures appears to have shifted from an earlier bemusement or indifference (combined with some irritation at the amount of time wasted) to a more recent positive enthusiasm for intervention. This outlook extends to patients (invariably, in my experience, fit young men) whose friends have had the full medical, but whose own employers do not stretch to the (considerable) expense. They turn up at the surgery, declaring that they 'need a complete checkup'. The popularity of the notion that healthy young people require regular medical maintenance marks the triumph of the ideology of health promotion.

As Bridget Jones also reflects, guilt is a more common response to health promotion initiatives than anger. When women have come in to the surgery worried about a breast lump, I have occasionally inquired whether they routinely carry out self-examination. The invariable response is 'No, but I know I should'. The fact that even people who do not follow the dictates of the 'awareness' campaigns – in this case into an activity which most experts consider quite useless – still feel that they are in default of their personal and social responsibilities, reveals the impact of health promotion. The gloomy atmosphere of the smokers' huddle confirms that who defy the injunctions of healthy living experience remorse rather than elation.

Over the past twenty years personal behaviour has been extensively re-interpreted and reorganised around considerations of health. The very ubiquity of terms which link 'health' with some activity which had previously been regarded as a distinct and autonomous sphere indicates this trend – 'healthy lifestyle', 'health foods', 'healthy eating', 'sexual health', 'exercise for health'. Whereas feminists once rejected 'women's health' as a form of male medical domination, their latter-day sisters have embraced 'lesbian health' as an affirmation of identity; in a common spirit of victimhood we now also have 'men's health'. The cult of exercise, pursued not for the enjoyment of sporting activity as such, but in the cause of improving physical fitness in the abstract, reflects the ascendancy of preoccupations about health over personal behaviour.

The third theme is the transformation of the medical role and the emergence of new institutions that mediate between the individual and the state in the sphere of health. The change in the role of the doctor is most apparent in general practice, in many ways the front line of the advance of medical intervention in lifestyle. In the not-so-distant past, general practice was a demand-led service: patients came to the surgery complaining of illness and doctors offered diagnosis and treatment, care and concern, within the limits of their own abilities and those imposed by medical science and health service resources. Over the past decade, general practice has shifted to a more pro-active approach, inviting patients to attend for health checks and screening procedures and adopting a more interventionist role in relation to lifestyle issues, such as smoking and drinking, diet and exercise. Instead of serving their patients' needs, GPs now serve the demands of government policy – and the dictates of government-imposed health promotion performance targets. New procedures, such as the routine check-up and the lifestyle questionnaire, allowing the systematic recording (now in a readily accessible computerised form) of intimate knowledge of the patient, have become a familiar feature of the doctor–patient relationship.

Having taken on a major role in health promotion, the government has worked with the established organisations of the medical profession – the various royal colleges, the BMA and others – to push forward initiatives like the *Health of the Nation* campaigns of the early 1990s. It has also recognised the limitations of these traditionally conservative and inflexible bodies and has encouraged the development of a range of institutions to play a more dynamic role. An early example of this approach was the establishment of the Health Education Council in 1968; this was transformed into the Health Education Authority in the heat of the Aids crisis twenty years later and was finally wound up in 2000 as its functions were subsumed by New Labour's Health Development Agency and other public health initiatives. The internal controversies of this body – and its well publicised tensions with government – reflect some of the difficulties involved in developing a novel health promotion approach (Farrant, Russell 1986). The anti-smoking campaign ASH, formed in 1971 with funding from the Department of Health, provided a model for numerous health-oriented voluntary organisations and pressure groups which flourished from the 1980s onwards, popularising health promotion messages. The big Aids charities – notably the Terrence Higgins Trust and the National Aids Trust – both heavily reliant on government funding, played a major role in the safe sex crusade. As we have seen, the big cancer charities have complemented the activities of the national screening agencies in encouraging women to have smears and mammograms.

Together with new health organisations and campaigns came a new corps of health professionals, skilled in the techniques appropriate to the advance of health promotion. Some of these were doctors, many more were nurses, only too keen to adapt their traditional skills to the requirements of the new discipline. While campaigning groups oriented towards politicians and the media required organisers, fund-raisers and journalists, those engaging with the public required skills in counselling in general, often combined with more specific expertise, required for example to give advice about diet, sexual behaviour or 'smoking cessation'. The exercise cult has provided employment for numerous personal trainers, aerobics instructors and others, who are now likely to have received basic health promotion training.

Health and morality

Has health become a new religion? The fact that activities once proscribed as sinful – gluttony, sloth, lust – are now regulated in the name of health has led numerous commentators to draw parallels between the ascendancy of health promotion over lifestyle today and the rule of religion in the past. The common features are indeed striking: the devotion to the cause of fitness displayed by the faithful, the spirit of self-denial required to sanctify the body, the zealotry of the newly converted, the dogmatism of the clergy. It appears that health provides some compensation for the decline of traditional religion, both as a focus of individual aspiration and as a secular moral framework for society.

The focus of health promotion on lifestyle risk factors for disease emphasises individual responsibility and demands compliance with the appropriate medically-sanctioned standard of behaviour as a duty to society. The burden of personal responsibility is reinforced by elevation of risks to others that may arise from individual failings: hence the emphasis on 'innocent victims' of HIV/Aids (children, haemophiliacs), the passive smoker, the foetus (of smoking, drinking, drug-taking mothers). Since traditional moral sanctions on behaviours considered deviant have become ineffective as a result of the declining power of the churches in society, values derived from health promotion have acquired growing influence. As the American historian Francis Fukuyama has noted, 'we feel entitled to criticise another person's smoking habits, but not his or her religious beliefs or moral behaviour' (quoted in Thomas 1997). Indeed smokers have become pariahs in modern society – and those who depart from other healthy lifestyle standards (such as the conspicuously obese) can also expect to meet with explicit social disapproval. In this way, the individual's state of health – as manifested in the state of their body – provides a sphere in which they can be held to account for their personal behaviour. People may no longer confess their sins to the priest in private, but their state of health provides public testimony to their conformity with the new moral code of healthy living, a code which is in many ways more authoritarian and intrusive than the religious framework it has replaced.

In expanding to fill the moral vaccuum resulting from the decline of the churches and the increasing fragmentation of society, medicine has come to play a much wider social role. It has displayed considerable flexibility in incorporating both traditional concerns about the decline of family values and fashionable commitments to pluralism and diversity, particularly in the sphere of sexuality. The philosopher David Mechanic has observed how medicine 'can be, at the same time, remarkably tolerant and extraordinarily judgemental', now accepting, for example, masturbation and homosexuality, after a long history of pathologising these activities, but fiercely condemning any departure from the safe sex code (Mechanic 1997). As Mechanic continues, there are such large areas of uncertainty today that 'moral entrepreneurs have endless opportunities to ply their trade'. Nowhere are these opportunities so great as they are in the sphere of health promotion.

It is important, however, not to exaggerate the potential of health to take over the role of religion. The parallels between Moses' Ten Commandments and Liam Donaldson's Ten Tips for Better Health are striking – they are even more explicit in the 'European Code Against Cancer, or Ten Commandments' cited in the *Health of the Nation* White Paper (DoH December 1999: xiv; DoH 1992: 66). But there are also significant differences. Injunctions against certain activities – 'thou shalt not' – are a feature of both codes, but figure even more prominently in the morality of health promotion. Whereas the Mosaic code emphasised the conduct of individuals in society, the healthy lifestyle commandments have a highly individualistic focus. As many commentators have noted, this narcissistic character of the contemporary cult of health reflects the anxieties of an increasingly atomised society. The fact, for example, that health promotion initiatives tend to be taken up more readily by the better off in society means that the advance of this agenda is likely to intensify social fragmentation rather than help to overcome it. Perhaps the greatest defect of health promotion, by contrast with traditional religion, is its lack of an inspirational element. Another version of the ten commandments of health promotion – the American Institute of Public Medicine's 'Ten New Year Resolutions' for 1992 – included alongside the familiar exhortations, recommendations to 'develop a social support network' and to 'have a sense of purpose' (quoted in Rosenberg 1997). If only tackling these great social and spiritual deficits of the late twentieth century Western world were as easy as other 'resolutions', such as 'avoiding second hand smoke' and 'limiting red meat, eggs and cheese'. Futhermore, when it comes to suffering and death, the inescapable elements of the human condition, the health promotionists fall silent.

While health promotion cannot replace religion, its moralism has a corrupting effect on medicine, as the American writer HL Mencken recognised in the 1920s:

> The aim of medicine is surely not to make men virtuous; it is to safeguard them and rescue them from the consequences of their vices. The true physician does not preach repentance; he offers absolution.
>
> (quoted in Skrabanek, McCormick 1989: 139)

5

THE POLITICS OF HEALTH PROMOTION

> The tidal wave of health promotion rhetoric seems, from my position in inner city general practice, to be an elaborate mechanism for blaming the victims.
> (Iona Heath, *The Mystery of General Practice,* 1995: 11)

The development of state-sponsored medical regulation of lifestyle in Britain was a prolonged and uneven process which may be divided into three more or less distinct phases. In the late 1970s, the Labour government first took up the cause of prevention, in a series of policy initiatives which made little immediate impact, but marked a significant innovation on which future policy-makers could build. A decade later, Margaret Thatcher's Conservative government launched what was claimed to be the biggest public health campaign in history in relation to Aids, and in the early 1990s extended its involvement in health promotion through the *Health of the Nation* initiative. After its election victory in 1997, New Labour appointed the first minister of public health and made the promotion of 'healthy living' a central theme of policy, not merely for the Department of Health, but for other government ministries. Looking at this period as a whole, the most striking features are the advance of state intervention in 'health-related' individual behaviour, the decline of critical responses and the absence of popular resistance. However, it is important to recognise that the process of state intervention in lifestyle advanced in fits and starts as a result of different government initiatives, driven by different concerns in different contexts and, in the early stages, with indifferent success. Let's take each phase in turn.

Blaming the victim

Given the major role the state currently occupies in health promotion, it is worth emphasising that this level of intervention in personal life is, apart from during war time, historically unprecedented. It is no doubt true that the reluctance of governments in the 1950s and 1960s to take action against tobacco in response to demands from medical bodies was largely attributable to fiscal and electoral considerations. Politicians at first rejected requests from anti-cholesterol campaigners to endorse their 'healthy diet' because of similar concerns about upsetting meat and dairy farmers, food processors and retailers – and their numerous and generally contented customers. Yet it would be a mistake to under-estimate the influence of popular traditions of suspicion of any official incursions on individual autonomy as a factor deterring state intrusion in individual behaviour, even in the cause of improving health. The greater vitality of such traditions in the USA explains the more intense controversy around these issues there compared with Britain where state intervention had become more widely accepted. However, even in Britain up to the 1960s there was some reticence among the medical elite about official intrusion into the personal domain. Thus, for example, the publication of the RCP's 1962 report recommending a public campaign against smoking followed an internal struggle of an incoming modernising leadership against an old guard personified by Lord Russell Brain, the eminent neurologist. Brain 'doubted very much' whether 'going beyond the facts' to 'giving advice to the public as to what action they should take in the light of the facts' should be the function of the college (Booth 1998).

The first major intervention of the state in health promotion came in the form of a discussion document produced under the authority of Labour health minister David Owen in 1976, entitled *Prevention and Health: Everybody's Business* (DHSS 1976). Its central theme was that 'much of the responsibility for ensuring his own good health lies with the individual' (DHSS 1976: 95). A White Paper, published the following year, with the same title, put the same message in a hectoring tone:

> Much ill-health in Britain today arises from over-indulgence and unwise behaviour. The individual can do much to help himself, his family and the community by accepting more direct responsibility for his own health and well-being.
>
> (DHSS 1977: 39)

In *Eating for Health* in 1979 the government claimed that an unhealthy lifestyle resulted from ignorance and irresponsibility and emphasised the need for information and education to change behaviour (DHSS 1979).

When Labour came to power in 1974, the country was in the grip of the recession that marked the end of the long post-war boom and its attendant social stability. At a moment when the government was preoccupied with the growing burden of public expenditure, Owen was appointed as a junior health minister. As a former hospital doctor, Owen was undoubtedly familiar with the radical critique of conventional medicine which had emerged over the preceding decade (see Chapter 8). He now adapted this critique to argue that 'preventive health measures' in relation to lifestyle could be an effective means of reducing health care costs (Owen 1976). A key influence on Owen was the innovative policy document produced by Canadian health minister Marc Lalonde in 1974, which recommended the pursuit of 'healthy public policies' by all government departments in support of the promotion of health (Lalonde 1974). While he recognised that 'government interference in all these areas raises sensitive issues relating to individual freedom' – a concern conspicuously lacking in more recent health promotion policy – Owen attempted to shift some of the responsibility, and cost, of health from the state onto the individual (Owen 1976).

In the inauspicious circumstances of the late 1970s, Owen's preventive strategy made little impact. He was an unpopular minister in an unpopular government: the wave of trade union militancy provoked by its wage controls and cuts in public expenditure culminated in the notorious 'winter of discontent' in 1978–79, which led directly to the election of Margaret Thatcher's first government in May 1979. As a result of a series of disputes over pay and private patients, the government had poor relations with the medical profession and, as an ambitious right-winger, Owen was regarded with particular suspicion by the unions (indeed he left Labour to set up the Social Democratic Party in 1981). Given the continuing strength of the collectivist traditions of the labour movement, the individualistic sentiments so bluntly expounded in Owen's documents found little popular resonance. In the USA, where government concerns with escalating health care costs were even greater than in Britain and trade unionism much weaker, the doctrine of individual responsiblity for health won greater approval (US Department of Health, Education and Welfare 1979, 1980).

Federal health promotion connected with a growing interest in self-help and consumerism, and with the vogue for jogging, marathon running and other forms of physical fitness, which reached Britain a few years later.

Government health promotion initiatives in the 1970s provoked a vigorous radical response, particularly in the USA. In a classic paper which anticipated subsequent trends with uncanny accuracy, the American sociologist Irving Zola commented that medicine was 'becoming a major institution of social control' (Zola 1972). He discerned a tendency towards the 'medicalising' of much of daily living which was proceeding in 'an insidious and often undramatic' way. Furthermore he noted that 'the list of daily activities to which health can be related is ever growing and with the current operating perspective of medicine it seems infinitely expandable'. As this process gathered momentum, the tone of the critique sharpened. In the late 1970s, another American sociologist, Robert Crawford, characterised health promotion as 'victim-blaming', an 'ideology which blames the individual for her or his illness and proposes that, instead of relying on costly and inefficient medical services, the individual should take more responsibility for her or his health. At-risk behaviour is seen as the problem and changing life-style, through education and/or economic sanctions, as the solution' (Crawford 1977). In his view, these 'ideological initiatives' had two functions. On the one hand, they served to 'reorder expectations and to justify the retrenchment from rights and entitlements for access to medical services'. On the other, they attempted 'to divert attention from the social causation of disease in the commercial and industrial sectors'.

The Health of the Nation

It was not until after her third general election victory in 1987 that Margaret Thatcher seriously set about reforming the health service. The 1989 White Paper *Working for Patients* heralded the introduction of the internal market into the NHS, with hospital trusts and GP fundholding. Yet, by the time these measures became operational in 1991, Mrs Thatcher had been replaced by John Major, and it was under his leadership that the *Health of the Nation* policy was introduced, with a Green Paper in June 1991 and a White Paper in July 1992 (DoH 1991, DoH 1992). This comprehensive health promotion programme was ideally suited to Major's attempt to project a more conciliatory 'one nation' Toryism in contrast to his predecessor's combative and divisive style. It also provided the perfect complement to the internal market reforms, appearing to soften their competitive edge while being quite consistent with their individualistic ethos.

A cursory inspection of the *Health of the Nation* package reveals that many lessons had been learned from Owen's ill-fated venture into health promotion in the 1970s. In his foreword to the Green Paper, health minister William Waldegrave indicated his concern to avoid criticism on the grounds of 'victim-blaming': 'for too long ... the health debate has been bedevilled by the two extreme claims of, on the one hand, "It's all up to individuals", and on the other, "It's all up to Government"' (DoH 1991: v). In what might be regarded as an early formulation of 'the third way', he insisted that 'we need a proper balance between individual responsibility and Government action'. The subsequent White Paper, presented by Waldegrave's successor Virginia Bottomley, continued this theme, emphasising that

> We must get the balance right between what the Government, and Government alone can do, what other organisations and agencies need to do and, finally, what individuals and families must contribute if the strategy is to succeed.
>
> (DoH 1992: 3)

The Conservative government had also clearly learned from Labour's earlier experiment that, if a policy directed at changing individual behaviour was going to make an impact on the public, it was necessary to foster intermediary institutions between the state and the people its policy was aiming to influence. The White Paper proposed a Cabinet-level coordinating committee and outlined specific roles for local authorities, the media, the Health Education Authority, and for employers and health professionals. It announced arrangements for providing funds for voluntary organisations, recognising that they could play a significant part through 'self-help', 'bringing people together to share common problems'; through 'direct service provision', offering a 'wide variety of services'; 'community health'; 'health education and promotion, education for health professionals, fund raising and support for research' (DoH 1992: 24–5). (This was particularly significant as it was virtually the only financial commitment in the document.) Furthermore, the White Paper emphasised the importance of promoting 'healthy alliances' among individuals and organisations working to fulfil the *Health of the Nation* strategy, and suggested a number of 'healthy settings' in which such alliances could operate, including 'healthy cities', 'healthy workplaces', 'healthy schools', 'healthy homes', 'healthy environments', even 'healthy hospitals' and, to make sure nobody was left out, 'healthy prisons'.

Though there were many differences between the circumstances in which the first two government initiatives in health promotion took place, one constant feature was the poor relations prevailing between the medical profession and the government. The internal market reforms presented in the 1989 White Paper were drafted without any consultation with doctors' leaders and in 1990 a new contract was imposed on GPs after it had been overwhelmingly rejected by GP representatives (Timmins 1995: 467). However, it rapidly emerged that, whatever the positions of their leaders, many doctors could see benefits in both hospital trusts and fundholding, and many GPs were keen to take advantage of the incentives offered by the new contract. Furthermore, some GPs who remained hostile to fundholding were keen on the preventive strategy advanced in the *Health of the Nation* documents and encouraged by the new contract. The endorsement by the BMA and the RCGP of a lavish *Health of the Nation* information pack, produced by the government and distributed free of charge to every GP, indicated the profession's general approval for the policy, whatever its past conflicts with the government.

Perhaps the most distinctive feature of the *Health of the Nation* policy was its identification of 'key areas for action' and its setting of precise targets in each of these areas. The five key areas were CHD and stroke, cancers, mental illness, HIV/Aids and sexual health, and accidents; the White Paper set fifteen targets in these areas and an additional ten 'risk factor' targets in matters such as smoking, diet and blood pressure. Though some of the targets – such as the aim to reduce the suicide rate by 15 per cent and the teenage pregnancy rate by 50 per cent by the year 2000 – provoked mockery, the very precision of the figures conveyed the seriousness of the government's commitment to its health promotion policy. Though this approach to defining objectives was widely criticised as a style of socialist planning, its inspiration came from the US health promotion policy introduced in the early 1980s, which had set 126 'achievable' objectives in reducing the burden of ill-health (US Department of Health, Education and Welfare 1980).

The *Health of the Nation* programme had a much greater impact than its predecessor. It is possible to evaluate the policy by placing a tick or a cross against each of its targets: thus death rates from CHD and stroke, and from breast cancer in women and lung cancer in men, fell to meet the targets (though cynics observed that they had been declining at this rate for some years), but rates of obesity and inactivity, teenage smoking, drinking among women and suicide among men, continued to rise (Calman 1998: 51). However, to judge the policy merely according to its own targets would be to underestimate its influence (Nuffield Institute for Health *et al.* 1998). Whether or not individual behaviour changed, the fact that, for example, in the course of the 1990s the smoker came to be regarded as a pariah, rather than as a person of coolness and sophistication, reflects the wider impact of the climate of opinion around issues of health that this policy did much to encourage. When a young woman said to me in the surgery 'I don't lead a bad life – I don't smoke, or drink much and I eat sensibly – so why do I feel ill all the time?' I recognised how widely and how deeply the message of the *Health of the Nation* had reached.

The greater impact of official health promotion propaganda in the 1990s compared with a decade earlier also revealed the enhanced sense of individual isolation that resulted from the Thatcher years. This was the result of a number of factors, including the persistence of mass unemployment and the resulting job insecurity and the increasing instability of family relationships. The breakdown of institutions and traditions of collectivity during the 1980s, best exemplified by the defeat and demoralisation of the trade unions, exacerbated the fragmentation of communities as well as labour movement organisations. The individuating dynamic resulting from unleashed market forces had destabilising consequences thoughout society, causing a heightened sense of personal vulnerability which often found expression in concerns about health.

The radical roots of health promotion

In her introduction to the *Health of the Nation* White Paper, Virginia Bottomley acknowledged the government's debt to the World Health Organisation's 'Health For All' strategy, noting that she 'was particularly heartened by the warm welcome which WHO gave' to the earlier Green Paper (DoH 1992: 2) This was a significant gesture of recognition to the deep roots of the *Health of the Nation* strategy in the radical critique of Owen's prevention policy in the 1970s. These roots can be traced through the activities of what became as the 'new public health' movement in international and domestic health agencies. As sociologist Sarah Nettleton has recognised, 'although health promotion and the new public health have now become incorporated into government health policies and mainstream health care, the concepts actually emerged from radical critiques of policies on the prevention of illness and 'conventional' approaches to health' (Nettleton 1995: 234).

The new public health movement was a product of the wider decline of the left. After a period of significant influence in Western societies from the late 1960s to the mid-1970s, the left subsequently experienced a series of defeats, culminating in its collapse following the disintegration of the Soviet bloc in 1989–90. One consequence of the disillusionment which had set in much earlier was the tendency for activists to retreat from public activity to attempt to pursue political objectives through their professional work, usually in some public service occupation, often in education or health. Though right-wingers often regarded 'the long march through the institutions' as a subversive strategy, it generally resulted in the abandonment of radical goals and, far from undermining the system, rather strengthened it with an infusion of youthful energy. Given the domination of national political life from the late 1970s onwards by the Conservative Party, many activists found alternative arenas which were much more open to their views in supra-national bodies like the European Community, the United Nations or the WHO, or alternatively, in local government. The beleaguered left-wingers refused to allow themselves to become further disheartened by the recognition that the openness of these bodies was in reality a result of their powerlessness. Nor did they pause to reflect that these international conferences were ready to approve radical resolutions because these resolutions had no practical consequences.

The key theme of the new public health movement was the need to shift the focus of health promotion from the level of the individual to tackle the wider social determinants of ill health (and unhealthy behaviour). The first triumph of the new public health took place at a conference organised jointly by the WHO and UNICEF in Alma Ata in what was then the Soviet Union in 1977. This conference adopted a declaration calling for 'Health For All', to be achieved 'by the year 2000' through a comprehensive programme amounting to the reconstruction of the world according to socialist principles of redistribution and equality. In 1985 the European office of WHO adopted a set of 38 targets against which progress of different national governments towards the goals of

'Health for All' could be measured. The 'new public health' made further advances the following year, when a conference in Ottawa endorsed the movement's emphasis on the 'empowerment' of communities to take the initiative in matters of health promotion away from governments and professionals. A further conference in Lisbon brought together new public health activists engaged in 'healthy city' projects organised by local councils, around the themes of 'equity in health', 'community participation', 'partnerships for health' and 'inter-sectoral collaboration'.

A number of critics have exposed the curious combination of utopian fantasy and cynical rhetoric that characterised the new public health movement. While activists projected a vision of revolutionary social transformation, it was only as employees of (decidedly moderate) government agencies that they had any prospect of implementing their health promotion policies. 'To state the matter baldly', as two disillusioned Canadian public health activists put it, 'the movement for health promotion is not a social movement but a bureaucratic tendency; not a movement against the state, but one within it' (Stevenson, Burke 1991).The Australian sociologist Deborah Lupton accurately identified a contradiction in the movement's conception of 'empowerment': if someone who is more powerful 'empowers' someone who is less powerful, their relationship is still didactic and paternalistic (Lupton 1995: 60). In a similar vein, Sarah Nettleton argued that the 'fallacy of empowerment' was revealed by the fact that health promotion was invariably oriented towards the least powerful people in society (Nettleton 1995: 238). A number of commentators noted the origins of the 'healthy cities' projects in 'paternalistic and cynical' 'community development' programmes developed by the British colonial office in the 1950s to contain potential unrest, suggesting that establishment concern about preventing inner city revolt after a series of riots in the early 1980s provided the impetus behind community health initiatives (Farrant 1991; Peterson, Lupton 1996). Critics also focused on the potential for discrimination and containment that lay behind concepts of 'community'. They observed that 'participation' often had a token character, which co-opted people into the existing power structure while giving them no real power in making decisions. Thus, while espousing a rhetoric of radical social change, in practice the activists of the new public health operated as professionals implementing government policies of an essentially conservative character.

While delegates to conferences in exotic international locations endorsed revolutionary declarations, supporters of the new public health at home sought to use these as a lever to press the government into adopting similar policies. A number of domestic influences, emerging more or less directly out of the experience of the previous Labour government, also encouraged the new public health movement.

The first was the controversy over 'health inequalities' that ran through the 1980s – and remains an issue under New Labour today. In response to growing concern among radical social policy academics about increasing income differentials and their impact on health under the Labour governments of the 1970s, in 1977 health minister David Ennals set up a working group chaired by Sir Douglas Black, president of the Royal College of Physicians. By the time the group had completed its report – in April 1980 – the government had changed and Mrs Thatcher was so hostile to the report's call for a redistribution of resources and a re-orientation of health services to tackle the problems of poverty that it was effectively suppressed (Black 1980). The resulting furore ensured an even bigger readership when *The Black Report* was briskly published by Pelican (Black 1982). It was re-issued in 1988, together with an extensive update by Margaret Whitehead and an introduction by two members of the original working group, as *Inequalities in Health* (Townsend, Davidson 1988). The issue of increasing inequalities in income and in indicators of health became a rallying cause for radical critics of the Conservative government in the 1980s, keeping ministers under pressure to bring forward some initiative in this area.

In the course of the 1980s a number of influential individuals and agencies encouraged the development of the government's health promotion policy. The chief medical officer Donald Acheson produced a report recommending an enhanced role for 'public health doctors' and also endorsed the WHO approach to monitoring progress in public health by setting targets (Acheson 1988). In 1985 the Kings Fund and the Health Education Council organised a 'study tour' to investigate health promotion in North America; a team closely identified with the new public health issued an enthusiastic endorsement of the WHO strategy on their return (Robbins 1987). The following year another multi-disciplinary committee sponsored by the Kings Fund, with the brief to chart progress since Owen's *Prevention and Health* in 1976, produced a report with the suggestive title *The Nation's Health* (Smith *et al.*

1988). This report also welcomed the WHO declarations and chastised the British government for its tardiness in meeting these targets. In its discussion of priority areas, strategies and targets, lifestyles and preventive services, it closely anticipated both the form and substance of the *Health of the Nation* documents. In the second 'new and completely revised' edition in 1991, the authors distinguished between the 'tradition of limited government responsibility for health and welfare' of which they disapproved, and the 'modern, international movement in public health' with which they strongly identified (Jacobson *et al.* 1991: 2). They further welcomed the emphasis on health promotion in the new GP contract, recognising that this offered 'new opportunities for developing public health practice'.

While key aspects of the new public health agenda attracted powerful supporters in the medical and political establishments, in 1987 its activists launched the Public Health Alliance as a new 'policy and pressure group'. Based in Birmingham, the alliance aimed 'to bring together voluntary and community groups, professional associations, local authorities, trade unions and individuals to promote and defend the public health in the UK' (Scott-Samuel 1989: 33). According to Alex Scott-Samuel, like most of the leading figures in the alliance a public health doctor, its most important goal was to make a reality of 'the principles behind the WHO Health For All strategy: the reduction of inequalities, intersectoral collaboration, primary health care and above all, community participation' (Scott-Samuel 1989: 35). The decisive weakness of the alliance resulted from the wider demise of the left: following the government's victory over the miners in 1984–85 and Labour's third consecutive general election defeat in 1987, left-wingers became increasingly isolated and marginalised in all areas of British society, including health. The resulting problem for the alliance's approach was that its aspirations for 'community participation' acquired the character of a fantasy, whereas the dependence of public health professionals on the state remained all too real. In practice, the radical ideals of 'Health For All' were rapidly subordinated to the pragmatic imperatives of government health policy.

The emergence of *The Health of the Nation* revealed the balance of forces determining public health policy and the limitations of the radical critique. Kenneth Clarke, as health minister, and Donald Acheson, as Chief Medical Officer, both encouraged the evolution of the Kings Fund's *The Nation's Health* into the government's *The*

Health of the Nation. In September 1991, following the publication of the Green Paper, the Public Health Alliance joined forces with the Radical Statistics Health Group in a conference to appraise the new policy (PHA 1992). In his introductory remarks, alliance chair Geoff Rayner welcomed the government's endorsement of health promotion and congratulated ministers for taking the 'first step' on a course which suggested a 'change of heart' following Mrs Thatcher's abrasive response to the Black Report. He hoped that the Green Paper might 'foreshadow a move away from a highly individualised, medicalised perspective on health' towards 'the philosophy of Health For All'. The main criticism advanced by Rayner and other speakers was that *The Health of the Nation* did not go far enough towards adopting the principles of the new public health, particularly on social inequality. Alex Scott-Samuel insisted that there was 'still a long way to go' before the government caught up with the objectives declared at the international conferences of the new public health.

Criticisms of the Conservative government for failing to adopt wholesale the radical programme of Alma Ata made little impact. Nobody expected a government that had made a principle of trying to destroy socialism suddenly to adopt a commitment to social equality in health or any other area. The government's interest in the new public health was not in its radical rhetoric, but in the potential of its health promotion policies to provide both a softer image for the Conservative Party and as mechanism for promoting greater individual responsibility for health. Hence it brushed aside calls for redistribution and for action against social causes of ill-health (such as unemployment, poor housing and the tobacco industry) and retained the familiar victim-blaming message of health promotion. Given the wider trends towards greater individuation in society, *The Health of the Nation* policy was inevitably experienced primarily as a campaign to change individual behaviour. In the absence of mass popular mobilisation against the state on any issue, continuing radical complaints that government health promotion emphasised individual behaviour instead of tackling social problems were more an expression of wishful thinking than a serious critique.

Health fascism?

While the left's critique of *The Health of the Nation* policy remained ineffectual, state health promotion encountered more substantial resistance from a group of doctors, academics and journalists loosely associated with the Social Affairs Unit, a right-wing think tank. By the end of the 1980s, the right, which had re-emerged a decade earlier to take advantage of the crisis of the left, was also in difficulties. Though the principles of privatisation and hostility for state welfare and trade unionism had encouraged the Thatcher project in its early years, the ideology of the free market had no answers for the renewed problems of recession in her third term and the growing crisis of government legitimacy. The exhaustion of conservatism was fully exposed when the end of the Cold War removed the focus – abroad and at home – that had given it cohesion and purpose for most of the century. However, whatever their wider problems, when confronted with the *Health of the Nation*, some conservative intellectuals retained sharper critical faculties than their erstwhile enemies on the left. The strengths of the right-wing critique of health promotion were its libertarian antipathy to state intrusion into personal life, its hostility to the moralising character of the new public health and its exposure of the junk science underlying it. The right's weaknesses lay in its inability to grasp the dynamic behind the government's health promotion policy and in its attempts to suggest an alternative approach.

The key figure in the critique of health promotion was Petr Skrabanek, a medical academic based in Dublin until his untimely death in 1994, who wrote a series of articles and essays which combined moral and intellectual force with wit and erudition. In his last book, published posthumously, entitled *The Death of Humane Medicine and the Rise of Coercive Healthism*, Skrabanek characterised 'healthism' as a repressive state ideology and 'Health For All' as a 'signpost on the road to unfreedom' (Skrabanek 1994: 11). He denounced politicians who indulged in the 'facile rhetoric of healthism' which 'increased their popularity at no cost' and 'enhanced their power to control the population' (Skrabanek 1994: 16). He reminded doctors that medicine was 'not about conquering diseases and death, but about the alleviation of suffering, minimising harm, smoothing the painful journey of man to the grave' (Skrabanek 1994: 22). He also reminded them that they 'had no mandate to be meddlesome in the lives of the well'. In his first book, written in collaboration with James McCormick and published only five year earlier, Skrabanek had challenged the notion of 'prevention as a crusade', which reminded him of 'the ideological simplicity of the quasi-religious crusades against the old enemies, sex, drugs, gluttony and sloth' (Skrabanek, McCormick 1989: 108). The authors condemned 'the self-righteous intolerance of some wellness zealots' with their policing of lifestyle, denial of pleasure and preaching of a modern form of asceticism. This vigorous defence of personal liberty against state coercion and professional puritanism stood in marked contrast to the left's casual endorsement of authoritarian health promotion policies (indeed radicalism on the left was measured by the scale of demands that the state go even further).

Skrabanek and his colleagues also advanced a devastating critique of the abuse of epidemiology and statistics by the advocates of the new public health. (Skrabanek, McCormick 1989; SAU/MI 1991). These publications clarified the confusions about association and causation, relative and absolute risk which, as we have seen, have played a major role in the rise of health promotion in relation to diet and CHD, passive smoking, and other controversies about risk factors and individual behaviour. They also exposed other examples of statistical scams and tendentious arguments used to justify interventions in lifestyle and screening programmes in relation to a wide range of diseases. The radical statisticians of the left identified so closely with the new public health movement that they were incapable of challenging the specious statistics on which much of the movement's policies were based.

Though the conservative critics of state health promotion provided a valuable service in challenging its authoritarian character and in exposing its cynical manipulation of epidemiology, their attempts to explain the origin of this policy were unsatisfactory and incoherent. Whereas Skrabanek denounced *The Health of the Nation* policy as 'health fascism', Bruce Charlton considered that it resembled 'a Soviet-style command economy'. The term 'health fascism' became popular in tabloid attacks on health promotion, which often focused on Virginia Bottomley who became something of a hate-figure for the Tory right. But Bottomley and Major seemed unlikely Nazis and the rhetoric of 'informed choice', 'non-judgemental' counselling and 'empowerment' that permeated official health promotion appeared far removed from the language of fascism. More importantly, though considered objectively *The Health of the Nation* had an authoritarian character, it was not perceived as coercive by the vast majority of people. The instinctive distaste for health promotion expressed by right-wing libertarians was understandable, but it also reflected their distance from the subjectivity of the British public.

Charlton's parallel between *The Health of the Nation* and Stalinist 'command and control' bureaucracy, with its plans and targets, had an immediate appeal (though Anderson's epithet 'food Leninism' seemed rather forced) (Anderson 1994). While conservative ideologues have never had difficulty in equating fascism and communism, they had a bigger problem reconciling the notion that the government had adopted a state socialist strategy towards health promotion at the very moment that its wider reforms of the health service were proceeding under the influence of an extreme version of the ideology of the free market, as expounded in *Working for Patients* (DoH 1989). As Charlton recognised, these appeared to be 'two distinct, and perhaps irreconcilable, philosophies of what the NHS is and what it should be' (Charlton 1994: 51). Behind *The Health of the Nation*, he discerned a 'peculiar alliance between the free marketeering right wing and the revolutionary left wing' (Charlton 1994: 55). Of course, no such alliance took place, not least because, by the early 1990s, both these familiar poles of twentieth-century politics had, for all practical purposes, ceased to exist. This made it quite possible for a pragmatic government to synthesise elements from different political traditions (an approach systematically pursued by New Labour under Tony Blair). Though in its twilight phase the Conservative government undoubtedly adopted some irrational measures (such as, for example, the Poll Tax), there was, as we have seen, a coherent thread running through its policies in the sphere of health.

In practice, there was no contradiction between *The Health of the Nation* and *Working for Patients*. The common theme of both documents was the promotion of individualism, in personal behaviour and in the provision of healthcare. Ironically there was more scope for this under the state-led health promotion policy than there was under the 'quasi-markets' in which competition between 'purchasers' and 'providers' was supposed to flourish. In these documents, which were both given high-publicity launches, style and symbol were as important as substance. In the *Health of the Nation*, socialist rhetoric provided a popular packaging for an essentially individualistic policy; in *Working for Patients*, free market rhetoric gave the impression of a more radical restructuring of the NHS than actually took place.

The problem was not the apparent contradiction between the two health White Papers, but the real contradiction between government aspirations for the emergence of a vibrant individualism and the fact that the individual who emerged from the ruins of the post-war welfare state was a conspicuously fragile person. The paradox of the new world order of the early 1990s was that, when the state had been rolled back and socialism crushed, the result was not a society of robust and intrepid entrepreneurs, but one of weak and vulnerable individuals. Instead of a climate of opinion which celebrated individual responsibility and autonomy, what emerged was a culture of complaint and victimhood, which elevated the values of safety over those of risk-taking, femininity over masculinity, childhood over adulthood (Furedi 1997). Just as the zest for privatisation turned into the pursuit of new forms of state support for faltering enterprise, so the 'empowerment' promised by health promotion led to the further medicalisation of personal life and the creation of new forms of dependency. And just as the level of state expenditure required to sustain private enterprise resisted all attempts at retrenchment, so, far from reducing health service spending, health promotion and the rising demands for reassurance it generated, drove costs further upwards.

Perhaps the greatest weakness of the right-wing critique of health promotion was its inability to explain the fact that, far from provoking public hostility to its intrusive and authoritarian measures, these were generally received with remarkable passivity, if not outright enthusiasm. The conservative critics advanced two complementary views. On the one hand they argued that the success of health promotion resulted from the more or less conspiratorial and manipulative activities of its propagandists. On the other, they attributed its impact to the climate of fear engendered in the public by health scares and panics. Skrabanek coupled these theses together in his argument that the popular preoccupation with risks to health was 'the result of a positive feedback between the masses stricken by fear of death and the health promotionists seeking enrichment and power (Skrabanek 1994: 38). He further commented that 'simple minds, stupefied by the sterilised pap of television and the bland diet of bowdlerised culture and semi-literacy, are a fertile ground for the gospel of the new lifestyle'. Though this revealed the author's patrician contempt for 'the masses', seriously compromising his claims to advance a humanist perspective, it did little to explain the rise of health promotion in the particular context of Western society in the 1990s.

The American neo-conservative theorist Irving Kristol advanced a novel sociological explanation for the influence of health promotion. He claimed that this was a result of the activities of a 'new class', which he freely admitted was 'a vague term', insisting that 'no useful purpose is served by trying to give it too precise a meaning' (Kristol 1994). His observation that 'one recognises its members when one sees them' suggested an appeal to the shared prejudices of his readers against people whose outlook was supposed to originate in the radicalism of the 1960s, and who now occupied prominent positions in the professions. Kristol believed that these people, with their unreconstructed anti-capitalist, pro-statist and environmentalist convictions, were now responsible for foisting health promotion on the people. It is true, as we have seen, that former radicals contributed much to the health promotion agenda, but this agenda was implemented in Britain by a government led by John Major, in which any trace of former long-hairs was difficult to discern.

Another theory, advanced by James LeFanu to explain the success of the diet-heart disease thesis, despite numerous studies which refuted it, was that its supporters had 'deliberately edited or censored evidence to justify their case' (LeFanu 1994). He attributed the triumph of the anti-cholesterol lobby in the USA in the early 1960s to the committee room intrigue of its leading advocates, which succeeded in winning the endorsement of the prestigious Americal Medical Association for a strategy of prevention based on recommending a 'healthy diet' (LeFanu 1999: 330–1). While these allegations may well be true, they do not explain either why similar policies were adopted in face of the evidence in other countries or why such policies have been so widely accepted by medical authorities, politicians and the public.

To turn to the public side of the manipulation of the masses thesis, references to a 'pervasive climate of cultural anxiety' are generally considered sufficient explanation for the popularity of health promotion initiatives (Berger 1994). The resonance for health scares has been variously attributed to fears of death and ignorance about science, but whereas these are scarcely novel phenomena, large scale panics about health are a development of the past decade. For some commentators, shifting attitudes on matters of health were simply changing fashions. Thus LeFanu explained the reversal of expert opinion on what constituted a healthy diet between the 1930s, when meat and dairy products were in favour, and the 1980s, when these were displaced by fruit and fibre, by the swing from '"high church" virtues of sensuousness and elitism' to '"low church" virtues of asceticism and egalitarianism' (LeFanu 1987: 158). But this elegant theory only shifted the problem elsewhere: how do we explain the shift in popular perceptions of virtue and their consequences for health?

The key defect of the right-wing critique of health promotion was its failure to grasp the dialectic between the state's resort to health promotion to compensate for its problems of legitimacy and the popular insecurities that had been generated by the social and political trends of the past decade, which found particular expression around issues of health. This interaction, facilitated by compliant doctors and operating through the medium of health promotion, between a state seeking authority and individuals seeking reassurance, provided enormous scope for government intervention in personal life and guaranteed the popularity of such intervention, however inadequate its scientific justification.

It is finally worth noting the fatalism of the right in what it regarded as a defensive, rearguard action against the advance of health promotion. As Kristol concluded gloomily, 'the laws have been passed, the institutions set up, the rules made: and I think our experience of the past ten years under quite conservative administrations indicates the difficulty of rolling back the wave' (Kristol 1994). When it came to policy alternatives to *The Health of the Nation*, the right-wing critics could only call for a return to old-style 'health education', with its explicit emphasis on individual responsibility (Anderson 1994). Not surprisingly, the right remained marginal and the health promotion wave kept on rolling.

Health inequalities and social exclusion

Tony Blair's New Labour government signalled its commitment to the cause of health promotion by immediately appointing Tessa Jowell as Britain's first minister of public health (though Yvette Cooper, who succeeded her in the October 1999 reshuffle, did not have a seat in the Cabinet). However, the subsequent policy documents revealed a high degree of continuity with *The Health of the Nation* policy (DoH December 1998, DoH July 1999). New Labour identified the same priority areas (though sexual health was hived off to a separate document), but cautiously reduced the number of targets to four – one in each area. In other respects the 1999 White Paper *Saving Lives* pushed forward along the same lines as the previous government (see Chapter One). To reflect the commitment of all relevant government departments to 'inter-sectoral collaboration' in the cause of health, the White Paper was signed by nine other ministers. It pursued the strategy of institutional innovation through its emphasis on 'health action zones', 'healthy living centres' and 'healthy citizens programmes' as well as by its endorsement of NHS Direct. And to confirm that the old 'victim-blaming' spirit was still thriving, *Saving Lives* opened by reminding readers that 'individuals too have a responsibility for their own health'.

The most significant difference from the past was that New Labour's health promotion initiative provoked virtually no opposition and very little criticism. The medical profession, which had been hostile to David Owen and ambivalent about Virginia Bottomley, greeted Tessa Jowell's policy with approval, if not enthusiasm. The only significant problems encountered by the government in this area resulted from external factors – its retreat on tobacco sponsorship of motor racing and a legal challenge to its attempt to ban cigarette advertising.

Saving Lives did focus on one subject that had been conspicuously avoided by the previous government – that of health inequalities. The White Paper emphasised that the government was 'addressing inequality with a range of initiatives on education, welfare-to-work, housing, neighbourhoods, transport and environment, which will help health' (DoH 1999: x) Critics pointed out that this wide range of government initiatives against inequality did not include the provision of higher levels of welfare benefits. The White Paper later asserted that 'the strong association between low income and health is clear' and immediately added that 'for many people the best route out of poverty is through employment' (DoH 1999: 45). For the many people for whom that route was not practicable, the White Paper offered no alternative. Given the continuing controversy around health inequalities, it is worth briefly tracing its evolution during the 1990s.

The concerns of the 1980s that increasing differentials in income were resulting in a growing gap between the health of the rich and that of the poor, became an increasingly prominent focus of medical research and discussion in the 1990s. Encouraged by Donald Acheson, the Kings Fund sponsored a series of investigations and seminars which culminated in the publication of *Tackling Inequalities in Health* in 1995, subtitled 'an agenda for action' (Benzeval *et al.* 1995). The BMA produced a report in the same year recommending a wide range of economic and social policies in response to this problem (BMA 1995). Both before and after its 1997 election victory, New Labour adopted the issue of health inequalities as one of its major themes, a preoccupation that is reflected in its public health policy documents.

At first inspection, the extent of medical and political concern with health inequalities appears puzzling. Though, as we have seen, class differentials have persisted, in real terms the health of even the poorest sections of society is better than at any time in history: indeed the health of the poorest today is comparable with that of the richest only twenty years ago (see Chapter One). Furthermore, it appears that the preoccupation with social class in the sphere of health (as indicated by the scale of academic publications) has grown in inverse proportion to the salience of class in society in general. After the emergence of the modern working class following the industrial revolution in the mid-nineteenth century, the question of class and its potential for causing social conflict and, for some, social transformation, dominated political life. It appears that after this era finally came to an end with the collapse of the Eastern bloc and the Soviet Union in 1989–90, and the political and social institutions organised around class polarisation lost their purpose, the subject suddenly became of much greater medical and academic interest. No longer subversive, class had acquired a new significance in relation to the social anxieties of the 1990s.

A closer examination of recent debates about issues of class and health reveals some of the concerns underlying the discussion of health inequalities. Whereas in the past the working class was regarded as the major source of instability in society, that menace has now receded, to be replaced by a perception of a more diffuse threat arising from trends towards social disintegration. The government's focus on issues such as crime and drugs, anti-social behaviour, teenage pregnancy and child poverty reflects its preoccupation with problems that appear to be the consequence of the breakdown of the family and of traditional communities and mechanisms for holding society together. All these concerns come together in the concept of 'social exclusion' which emerged in parallel with increasing concerns about health inequalities. At the launch of the Social Exclusion Unit, a key New Labour innovation, in December 1997, Tony Blair summed up the significance of the concept for New Labour: 'It is a very modern problem, and one that is more harmful to the individual, more damaging to self-esteem, more corrosive for society as a whole, more likely to be passed down from generation to generation, than material poverty' (*The Times*, 9 December 1997). The term social exclusion appears to be less pejorative and stigmatising than more familiar notions such as 'the poor' or 'the underclass'. Social exclusion also implies a process rather than a state: people are being squeezed out of society, not just existing in conditions of poverty. It expresses a novel sense of guilt over the failures of society as well as the familiar condescension towards the poor. Above all it expresses anxiety about the consequences of social breakdown as well as fear of crime and delinquency.

The concepts of equality and inequality have also undergone a significant re-interpretation. This began with the Commission on Social Justice, a think-tank set up in 1992 in the inter-regnum between Neil Kinnock and Tony Blair, when John Smith was Labour leader; it reported in 1994 after his sudden death (Commission on Social Justice 1994). After Labour's fourth and most bitter election defeat, this body accelerated the process of ridding the party of its social democratic heritage that had begun under Kinnock and was completed under Blair. It shifted Labour's goal from social equality to social justice, which it defined as recognition of the 'equal worth' of all citizens (CSJ 1994: 18). In place of the traditional view of inequality as a question of the distribution of the material resources of society, the commission explained it in cultural and psychological terms. Thus it emphasised that 'self respect and equal citizenship demand more than the meeting of basic needs; they demand opportunities and life chances'. It concluded that 'we must recognise that although not all inequalities are unjust ... unjust inequalities should be reduced and where possible eliminated'. Once Labour had accepted Mrs Thatcher's famous dictum 'Tina' – 'there is no alternative' to the market – then it had also to accept the inevitability of inequality. Its traditional clarion call to the cause of equality gave way to feeble pleas for fair play.

In his emotional speech to Labour's centenary conference in September 1999, Tony Blair reaffirmed the government's commitment to tackling inequalities in British society and pledged to 'end child poverty within a generation'. While this went down well with party traditionalists, Blair was careful to put the distinctive New Labour spin on the concept of equality. Thus he reaffirmed that, for New Labour, 'true equality' meant 'equal worth', not primarily a question of income, more one of parity of esteem. As Gordon Brown put it, poverty was 'not just a simple problem of money, to be solved by cash alone', but a state of wider deprivation, expressed above all in 'poverty of expectations'. In case there was any misunderstanding, Anthony Giddens, chief theoretician of the third way, bluntly explained that there was, 'no future' for traditional left-wing egalitarianism and its redistributionist 'tax and spend' fiscal and welfare policies (Giddens 1999). Instead 'modernising social democrats' needed 'to find an approach that allows equality to coexist with pluralism and lifestyle diversity'. Giddens' new egalitarianism meant accepting wide differentials in income, but insisting on 'equal respect'. New Labour's message to the poor was: never mind the width of the income gulf – feel the quality of our recognition of your pain.

A continuing tension between Old and New Labour approaches to inequality was also apparent in the health inequalities debate. For one group of traditionalists, based in Bristol, 'poverty really is a problem of the lack of enough money – if you give poor people enough money they stop being poor – it is as simple as that' (Shaw *et al*. 1999: 184). For Richard Wilkinson at Sussex University, a prominent figure in this debate over two decades, it was not so simple. He maintained that social differentials in health were the result of 'psychosocial' rather than material factors, as the 'chronic stress' generated by a polarised society takes its toll on the health of those who are relatively worse off (Wilkinson 1996: 214–15). Whereas the Bristol group insisted that 'poverty reduction really is something that can be achieved by "throwing money at the problem"', Wilkinson argued that the solution lay in strategies to 'achieve narrower income distribution and better social cohesion' (Shaw *et al*. 1999: 191; Wilkinson 1996: 222). In the harsh world of politics, New Labour's slavish devotion to Tina, fiscal rectitude and electoral expediency mean that it has no intention, either of raising benefits to the poor, or of doing anything to reduce income differentials. The Bristol group's repeated demands that such measures 'should be their top priority' in face of the unmistakable evidence that government policy is moving in the opposite direction reflect the pathological dependence of Old Labour on New Labour, like that of the battered wife who cannot abandon her abusive partner. Yet, while the government is doing nothing to reduce income differentials, it is very active around issues of health inequalities and social exclusion.

Back in 1995 the Kings Fund 'agenda for action' against health inequalities indicated four levels of policy intervention:

- strengthening individuals;
- strengthening communities;
- improving access to essential facilities and services;

- encouraging macroeconomic and cultural change.

(Benzeval *et al.* 1995: 24)

Interventions at level four were of the character of WHO declarations, worthy statements of principle and sentiment, without practical consequences. Level three interventions concerned attempts to promote collaboration in the cause of health among government departments responsible for areas such as employment, housing, education and welfare. Thus, for practical purposes, tackling inequalities in health was a question of individual and community initiatives.

Policy responses at the first level were 'aimed at strengthening individuals in disadvantaged circumstances, employing person-based strategies' (Benzeval *et al.* 1995: 25). Examples provided included 'stress management education for people working in monotonous conditions, counselling services for people who become unemployed to help prevent the associated decline in mental health and supportive smoking cessation clinics for women with low incomes'. According to David Wainwright's perceptive critique of this report, 'the objection should not be that such initiatives *blame* the individual, but that they reinforce his/her low expectations concerning social change' (Wainright 1996). Furthermore, 'by encouraging the individual to adapt to adverse conditions, to be a "survivor", such initiatives reinforce the belief that any form of social action is unlikely to succeed, that one should just accept one's alienation'. He challenged the notion that using such 'cheap psychological tricks' could contribute to 'empowerment', observing that the 'colonisation of the individual's life-world' involved in these schemes was the 'ultimate in *dis*empowerment'.

Policies aimed at the level of the community were 'focused on how people in disadvantaged communities can join together for mutual support and in so doing strengthen the whole community's defence against health hazards' (Benzeval *et al.* 1995: 25). The first three targets proposed for community mobilisation were as follows:

- social control of illegal activity and substance abuse;
- socialisation of the young as participating members of a community;
- limiting the duration and intensity of youthful 'experimentation' with dangerous and destructive activity

Though it is not at all clear how such initiatives would reduce health inequalities, the attempt to use policies presented in the guise of health promotion as a means of social control is obvious. Tackling health inequalities has become redefined as community policing to deal with problems of drugs, crime and even youthful exuberance (now known as 'anti-social behaviour'). The authors' statement that 'these policies recognise the importance to society of social cohesion, as well as the need to create the conditions in deprived neighbourhoods for community dynamics to work' provides considerable insight into their own preoccupations (which are no doubt widely shared in the medical and political establishments).

Since the election of New Labour to government and the elevation of health inequalities and social exclusion to the centre of policy, interventions targeted at individuals and communities of the sort earlier promoted by the Kings Fund have become commonplace. In an updated set of recommendations, Michaela Benzeval and her colleagues suggested, as one example of an initiative to combat health inequalities, 'home visiting by health visitors, GPs and trained community peers to reinforce preventive health measures' (Benzeval, Donald 1999: 94). How would one conduct such a 'reinforcement' visit? Confiscate cigarettes, count up household alcohol units and dispose of any excess to basic weekly requirements, inspect the fridge for high fat foods and confiscate cream buns, organise a brisk jog around the block? The activities of the Social Exclusion Unit around issues like homelessness and teenage pregnancy do nothing to reduce inequality, but aim to foster a therapeutic relationship between the state and recipients of welfare benefits. Programmes like Sure Start, which aims to promote the parenting skills of young families also aim to provide new points of contact between isolated individuals and the state. Meanwhile the activities of health action zones and healthy living centres also aim to foster the social cohesion for which New Labour yearns. Under the banner of health inequalities New Labour has turned health promotion into a sophisticated instrument for the regulation, not only of individual behaviour, but that of whole communities.

6

THE EXPANSION OF HEALTH

Over the past decade GPs have moved away from their traditional commitment to the individual patient to take on a wider role in tackling the problems of society. The treatment of drug addicts is one example of this trend, which is leading to a transformation in the nature of medical practice as GPs take on some of the concerns of the criminal justice system. The expanding scope of general practice extends into the field of mental health, a territory that has itself expanded through the annexation of more and more areas of personality and behaviour under psychiatric disease labels. We focus here on the expansion of the concept of addiction and at the way this has contributed to the growing medicalisation of society. We look finally at the treatment of these problems in general practice, through counselling and medication and at the consequences of these developments for both doctors and patients.

Drug squad general practice

In the 1980s and early 1990s I gained some experience in the medical approach to treatment of drug addiction in general practice. The occasional heroin user would turn up, usually in a stereotypically 'strung-out' condition, saying that they wanted to come off drugs and asking for a prescription for methadone. Following the approach recommended in various text-books and official publications, I would try to assess their motivation to get off drugs and if this seemed positive, I would agree to prescribe methadone and refer them to the drug dependency unit at the local hospital, for specialist counselling (Advisory Council on the Misuse of Drugs, 1982, 1984). I would work out how much heroin they were using and calculate the appropriate dose of methadone and negotiate a programme of withdrawal over a period of weeks or months, according to what appeared realistic. We would then arrange to meet weekly to renew prescriptions and review progress.

My experience of this technique over several years was of approximately 100 per cent failure. Sometimes the withdrawal programme appeared to be going well for while, but then things would start to fall apart. Sometimes the patient simply disappeared, only to return months later, even more strung-out, wanting to start the whole process again. Sometimes they would turn up, invariably late and often in an agitated state, with a variety of explanations often of remarkable ingenuity, which all culminated in a demand, more or less aggressively delivered, for further prescriptions of methadone or other medications. Sometimes they would reach the end of the withdrawal phase and simply request to continue on a substantial dose of methadone into the indefinite future. Reflecting on this experience, I recognised two fundamental problems with the substitute medication approach, one relating to motivation, the other to addiction. It became clear that assessing motivation was superfluous because the very fact that somebody presents their drug problem to a GP in the form of a request for methadone confirms that their motivation is to continue rather than to stop taking drugs. They simply want to continue in a different way, getting less of a high perhaps, but also getting less hassle. The high level of conflict between GPs and drug users arises from this basic confusion: while the GP thinks they want to stop, the user just wants to continue.

Bob Scott, clinical director of the Glasgow Problem Drug Service, acknowledged this point in a thoughtful contribution to a conference on managing drug users in general practice (Scott 1997). He observed that when patients were asked what their expectations of treatment were, 'almost without exception they stated that the principal reason for approaching services was to obtain "help"'. However, 'on gentle probing, "help" always meant a prescription for a controlled drug'. He could recall nobody saying that they expected to improve their health and only one person who wanted to become drug-free in order to look for work. While Dr Scott emphasised the need to acknowledge and reconcile these conflicting expectations, I began to question the whole policy of substitute medication.

The second problem follows from the endorsement of the concept of addiction. Whereas heroin is generally considered to be highly addictive, methadone is not. Yet people who consider themselves addicted to heroin are quite capable of becoming addicted to methadone, or even relatively minor analgesics like dihydrocodeine or coproxamol, which are not regarded as addictive and have only slight narcotic effects. This suggests that the pattern of behaviour associated with drug addiction is socially conditioned rather than being biologically or pharmacologically determined.

When I come across people who have taken drugs like heroin in the past, sometimes for quite long periods, I often ask them what made them stop. It turns out that this is rarely the result of drug treatment programmes, 'detoxification' or 'rehabilitation', but usually follows some wider change of lifestyle prompted by a new partner or a new job, a spell in prison or by simply getting bored with the drug scene. This confirms that when people really decide to stop, they just stop and often report relatively little difficulty in overcoming the much-publicised problems of physical and psychological dependency. Though the official drug misuse guidelines emphasise that methadone prescription 'should be seen as an enhancement to other psychological, social and medical interventions', I have become increasingly sceptical about the value of these initiatives.

Methadone maintenance

At the very time, in the mid-1990s, that I was coming to the conclusion that prescribing methadone was not a useful way of treating drug addicts, GPs came under renewed government pressure to participate in a more comprehensive drug treatment programme. The sequence of events leading up to the current large scale prescribing of methadone in general practice reflects not only a significant change in the management of drug abuse, but also a transformation in the nature of general practice. The government White Paper *Tackling Drugs to Build a Better Britain*, published in 1998, and the 'guidelines on clinical management' published the following year, proclaimed the leading role of GPs in managing drug abuse and the virtues of 'methadone maintenance treatment' (President of the Council 1998; DoH 1999). This marked a significant shift away from the earlier strategy of encouraging GPs to refer drug addicts to specialist centres. It also reflected the ascendancy of what has been dubbed the 'public health' approach to drug abuse over a 'client or patient-centred' approach.

In the past, the straightforward objective in treating heroin addicts was to get them off drugs. Methadone was developed in Germany during the Second World War as a pain-killer. It does not have the euphoric effects of heroin, but blocks the adverse effects of heroin withdrawal. It also has the advantages that it has a longer duration of action (and can therefore be taken as a daily dose) and can be taken by mouth (rather than by injection). Since its introduction into the treatment of heroin addiction in the USA in the 1940s it has been prescribed to patients in steadily reducing doses, with a view to achieving abstinence.

The new 'public health' approach has largely abandoned the goal of abstinence in favour of 'harm reduction'. The objective is no longer to make the heroin user drug free, but to replace dependence on heroin with long-term dependence – 'maintenance' – on methadone. The aim is that this should in turn reduce reliance on illicit drug supplies, curb needle-using and needle-sharing and, above all, curtail the criminal activities that may be required to raise the funds necessary to sustain a heroin habit. The main concern of this policy is not the welfare of the individual drug user, but the stability and security of society. If we look back to the previous edition of government guidelines, published in 1991, the change in approach is striking (DoH 1991). This document outlines a range of patterns of prescribing, including 'rapid withdrawal', 'gradual withdrawal' and 'maintenance-to-abstinence (long-term with-drawal)' (DoH 1991: 22). It also refers cautiously to 'maintenance (stabilisation)', a policy of 'indefinite' prescription with 'no immediate intention of withdrawal', as one which 'has been suggested' and which may be a 'helpful approach' for a 'small proportion of patients'. However, the document continues, 'it is not described further here as it is a specialised form of treatment best provided by, or in consultation with, a specialist drug misuse service'. Yet it is this approach which has, within a decade, become the dominant form of drug treatment in general practice.

The 1991 document did, however, indicate the shift towards 'harm minimisation' as the goal of medical intervention. The key factor here was the advent of Aids and fears that needle sharing might facilitate the spread of HIV infection. As a BMA guide later explained, 'prescribing was no longer solely aimed to help the drug user become drug free', but had become 'a useful tool in the prevention of HIV spread' (BMA 1997: 11). A new hierarchy of 'aims of harm minimisation' was declared:

- stop or reduce use of contaminated injecting equipment
- stop or reduce sharing of infected equipment
- stop or reduce drug misuse

(DoH 1991: 18)

This policy of prescribing 'primarily for public health reasons to prevent the spread of HIV out into their local general heterosexual community', as the BMA put it, 'and only secondarily to help drug users address their drug problem' became 'the mainstay of treatment policy' (BMA 1997: 11). Nevertheless, it is worth noting that, in a 'schematic presentation of the assessment and management of a drug problem' in the 1991 document, the box 'DRUG FREE' is the target towards which all the arrows point (DoH 1991: 12).

Joining the Drug Squad

By the mid-1990s the panic about Aids had subsided, and there was a resurgence of public fears about crime, increasingly linked by politicians and in the media, to drugs. As a result, the public health approach to drug misusers was increasingly supplemented by a criminal justice approach. The interests of the individual patient receded even further from the centre of attention.

The 1995 White Paper *Tackling Drugs Together* emphasised the link between drugs and crime. It set up local 'drug action teams' bringing together senior figures from health and local authorities with representatives of the police and the probation and prison services. This document offered a 'statement of purpose' and a new hierarchy of goals:

> To take effective action by vigorous law enforcement, accessible treatment and a new emphasis on education and prevention to:
>
> - increase the safety of communities from drug-related crime;
> - reduce the acceptability and availability of drugs to young people; and
> - reduce the health risks and other damage related to drug misuse.
>
> (President of the Council *et al.* 1995)

Doctors were coming under increasing pressure to participate in a 'multi-agency' and 'shared-care' approach to drug misuse, guided by a policy in which the first priority was to reduce crime. Given the central commitment of the government to 'vigorous law enforcement', it was not surprising to find that the interests of the misuser came a poor third.

The commitment to reduce drug-related crime was a central theme in the 1998 White Paper which, by offering cash incentives to GPs to take on methadone prescribing, proved the decisive stimulus to the expansion of this programme. Yet the link between drugs and crime remains controversial. An earlier Scottish Office inquiry commented that it was 'highly doubtful' whether an accurate mechanism could be devised for recording drug-related crime' (BMA 1997: 49). The BMA's judgement was that 'until more research is conducted on the "drugs-crime" connection, all that can be said is that drugs and crime are associated in some way for some individuals' (BMA 1997: 49). A later review of the literature concluded that 'the empirical evidence does not support' the belief that drug addiction is the motor behind much property crime in Britain (Seddon 2000). The author warned that 'drug treatment as a panacea for property crime is a strategy unlikely to succeed'. Yet despite the lack evidence for the drug-crime link, this has remained the dominant justification for government policy.

The White Paper provided a revealing example of anti-drugs policy-making. Emphasising the importance of basing strategy on evidence, it quoted the 'latest indications from a random sample of suspected offenders arrested by the police suggest that over 60 per cent of arrestees have traces of illegal drugs in their urine' (President of the Council 1998). Though this evidence was widely reported in the media, a response, which pointed out that it was 'based on shaky ground if we examine the report from which it is derived', was not (Stimson *et al.* 1998). The samples were taken at three sites chosen for convenience (Hammersmith, Manchester and Cambridge); they were not taken at random and, in more than 40 per cent of those found to be positive, tests revealed only cannabis – which can show traces in urine for up to one month. In other words, this study showed that quite a few people arrested in inner city areas may have smoked a joint in the previous few weeks. Though, as Stimson *et al.* pointed out, the author of the study was cautious in interpreting the results of a preliminary investigation, the government manipulated this research to justify its anti-drugs policy.

A similarly low level of scientific rigour is apparent in the claim by promoters of the new drug policy that there is 'strong evidence for the effectiveness of methadone maintenance treatment' (Keen 1999). In fact, this demonstration of the effectiveness of methadone has been achieved by moving the goal posts. Recognising the ineffectiveness of using reducing doses of methadone to achieve the traditional goal of abstinence, its supporters now claim that methadone maintenance is successful in reducing the wider damaging consequences of heroin use. In fact, some evidence suggests that it is most successful in reducing 'drug-related criminal behaviours', less so in reducing illicit opiate use and even less so in reducing 'risk behaviours' associated with the transmission of hepatitis or HIV (Marsch 1998).

The preliminary results of the major research programme sponsored by the Department of Health (National Treatment Outcome Research Study) similarly claim success on a variety of outcome measures, though not that of enabling the user to become drug free (Glossop *et al.* 1999). Researchers found that, after six months on methadone programmes (either in GP surgeries or specialist clinics), users had achieved a significant reduction in the use of heroin and other illicit drugs and a lower rate of injecting. It is scarcely surprising that if users are provided with opiates by doctors, their use of illicit opiates declines. The survey also claimed an improvement in physical health, reduced levels of depression – and reduced rates of non-drug-related crime.

The BMA report emphasises the limitations of British evidence to date and the fact that much of the evidence guiding policy in Britain is derived from the USA (BMA 1997: 76). The problem here is not only the difference of context, but that the American evidence is also disputed. Sociologist James Nolan has conducted a detailed study of the results of the Dade County Drug Court in Florida, the model for drug treatment programmes in the USA and beyond. He notes that while 'initial findings regarding recidivism rates appear fairly impressive' – particularly when conducted 'in-house' – 'studies conducted by agencies outside the Drug Courts, however, are less encouraging' (Nolan 1998: 104). Reviewing the figures and revealing various statistical scams, Nolan wonders whether 'such liberty in adjusting measurements would explain the discrepancy between the low recidivism rates reported by the courts … and the much higher rates found by external agencies?' (Nolan 1998: 109). He also notes a tendency to adopt different measures of outcome, replacing the goals of staying off drugs and away from crime, with an acceptance of reports of participation and progress in therapy as positive indicators. His conclusion from careful examination of the conviction that drug treatment 'works', is that 'it appears that the more subjective, emotive perspective has super-seded, or at least redefined what is meant by "it works"' (Nolan 1998: 112).

Does drug treatment cut crime? Further evidence is presented in a paper entitled 'Can methadone maintenance for heroin-dependent patients retained in general practice reduce criminal conviction rates and time spent in prison?' (Keen *et al.* 2000). This study examined the criminal records of 57 patients in maintenance methadone programmes at two general practices in Sheffield. It claims to show that they had significantly fewer convictions and spent significantly less time in prison after they started on methadone. However, it reports the decline in convictions and time in prison only in relative terms, making it impossible to judge its real significance. But the more important issue is whether the question posed in the title of the paper is a legitimate concern for general practice. Is it my job as a GP to cut crime? Keeping people out of court and out of prison may be a laudable objective for society as a whole, and it is an understandable concern for those involved in the criminal justice system. But it has never before been regarded as a goal of medical practice.

Methadone: an ethical imperative?

What about the patient? There is no doubt that methadone is less damaging to health than injecting heroin: apart from the risks associated with acquiring illicit drugs, there are dangers of overdose and contamination, and the spread of a wide range of infections, most significantly hepatitis B and C. (For various reasons, HIV has never reached a high prevalence among drug abusers in Britain, though some localised epidemics have occurred, notably in Edinburgh.) However, methadone is not without its own dangers. The most familiar side-effects are drowsiness and constipation, but it can also cause urinary problems, dry mouth, sweating, facial flushing, vertigo, palpitations, slow pulse rate and mood changes. Furthermore there are serious risks of overdose, which causes low blood pressure and suppresses respiration.

There have been reports of an increased number of deaths from methadone (which now exceed those from heroin). A survey in Manchester revealed 90 deaths from methadone between 1985 and 1994, with a dramatic increase following the introduction of methadone maintenance programme in 1990, a pattern that is reflected nationally (Cairns *et al.* 1996). Another report from Lothian indicated that deaths from methadone more than doubled between 1995 and 1996 (Greenwood *et al.* 1997). Furthermore, a large proportion of these deaths occurred in individuals who had not been prescribed methadone, confirming the diversion of prescribed methadone into the illicit drug market. A survey on Merseyside reported 44 accidental overdoses of methadone among children and two deaths (Binchy *et al.* 1994). Following the death of a three-year-old boy in Dublin who accidently consumed methadone kept by his parents (for measuring purposes) in a baby's bottle, a survey revealed this to be a widespread practice (the Manchester figures included four fatalities among young children) (Harkin *et al.* 1999).

Despite the evidence of the dangerous consequences of methadone for individual drug users and their families, the pressures on GPs to participate in methadone maintenance have intensified. In East London, we have been bombarded with methadone propaganda and invited to specially organised local seminars. The new guidelines are linked with cash incentives, offering GPs around £20 per month per patient. More ominously, with the carrot comes the stick. An editorial in the *BMJ*, significantly written by the main author of the Sheffield study quoted above, after asserting that the efficacy of methadone maintenance 'is now so well established' inquired rhetorically: 'for how long can it be considered ethical for some GPs to refuse to prescribe it within a shared care framework?' (Keen 1999). Such is the degradation of medical ethics that it is now considered virtuous for doctors to take on the role and responsibilities of the police and to subordinate the best interests of their patients to the dictates of government drug policy. Is it now to be considered ethical for GPs to take on the role of the police in relation to their patients?

In his comprehensive history of modern medicine, Roy Porter comments caustically on the way in which, in the 1940s, 'the American medical profession fell into line with the criminalisation of narcotics, accepting funds made available for setting up detoxification units and the development of anti-addiction drugs like methadone' (Porter 1997: 666). Though Porter confines his censure of the medical profession to the past, his criticism of the US physicians of the 1940s has a remarkable contemporary resonance: 'They could easily convince themselves that they were helping addicts and society, while doing their careers a favour'.

When drug addicts ask for methadone today, I try to explain the conclusions I have drawn from my experience and my particular reluctance to play the role of a deputy constable in the drug squad in the current methadone programme. If they still want methadone, I refer them to the appropriate local agency. Otherwise, I indicate that I would be happy to help them with their general medical problems, while leaving their drug problem to the only person competent to sort it out, themselves. I find that this approach opens the way to a much more constructive doctor–patient relationship than I could ever achieve while haggling over doses of methadone.

The devaluation of diagnosis

You meet a lot of people in general practice who defy conventional psychiatric categories, but who are equally clearly some way beyond the realm of any concept of normality. There are some people whose personality seems so eccentric and whose ways of thinking and speaking are so bizarre that you sometimes wonder how they survive in a world that requires considerable skills of coping and survival. But, in their own ways, they do. You also meet a lot of unhappy people, indeed by Friday evening you would readily agree with H.D. Thoreau that many, if not most, people 'lead lives of quiet desperation' (Thoreau 1854: 50). In some their distress is expressed in physical symptoms, of total body pain or feeling tired all the time; in others it is openly proclaimed as sadness, loneliness or rage.

In John Berger's celebrated 'story of a country doctor', he wrote that the task of the doctor when confronted with an unhappy patient offering an illness was to recognise the person behind the illness (Berger, Mohr 1967: 69). This act of recognition itself can help to overcome hopelessness and even begin to offer 'the chance of being happy'. To make an unhappy person feel recognised, the doctor 'has to be oblique' and yet has to appear to the patient as a comparable person, a process which demands 'a true imaginative effort and precise self-knowledge'. This well captures the challenge of general practice.

'The whole process' of recognition, observed Berger, 'as it includes doctor and patient, is a dialectical one'. The doctor must recognise the patient as a person, but for the patient, 'the doctor's recognition of his illness is a help because it separates and depersonalises that illness'. This is why, he continued, 'patients are inordinately relieved when doctors give their complaint a name'. Even if the name means little, it gives their condition an independent existence: 'they can now struggle or complain *against* it'. For the patient to have a complaint 'recognised', in the form of a diagnosis which is 'defined, limited and depersonalised ... is to be made stronger'. Reading Berger's account more than thirty years after it was written, we can still appreciate the importance he placed on recognition. What has changed is the healing power of diagnosis: we can no longer claim that giving the patient a name for their illness makes them stronger, even if it may still give them some relief. If we look, concentrating on the sphere of psychiatry, at the three features of the diagnosis that he considered gave people strength to deal with their afflictions, major changes are apparent.

Whereas in the past mental illnesses were few and clearly defined, today disease labels are both more numerous and more diffuse. In 1952, the *Diagnostic and Statistical Manual* of American psychiatry recognised 60 categories of abnormal behaviour; by 1994 this had expanded to 384 (plus 28 'floating' diagnoses) (American Psychiatric Association 1994). Furthermore psychiatric authorities have identified a much wider prevalence of 'sub-syndromal behaviour'. Some reckon that many, if not most, people in society are suffering from 'shadow syndromes', mild or partial forms of familiar psychiatric conditions, such as depression and anxiety, obsessional compulsive disorder and autism (Ratey, Johnson 1997). Clinical psychologist Oliver James, author of the popular book *Britain on the Couch*, snappily subtitled 'why we're unhappier compared with 1950 despite being richer: a treatment for the low-serotonin society', reckons that around one third of British adults could be diagnosed as having some form of 'psychiatric morbidity' (James 1997: 307). Adding those manifesting tendencies towards 'violence and aggression' brings the proportion of those deemed in need of intervention 'to around one half – perhaps twenty million people' (James 1997: 308–9).

At the time that Berger wrote, there was a general inclination to emphasise the discontinuity between the normal and the abnormal; today the concept of a continuum has become fashionable. The invention of new disease labels – such as 'attention deficit hyperactivity disorder' in children or diverse forms of addiction in adults – reflects the trend to define a wider range of experience in psychiatric terms. It also results in a further blurring of the boundary between the normal and the abnormal. Whereas diagnoses previously suggested the limited character of the condition, modern disease labels imply disorders that are unrestricted in the scope of the symptoms to which they give rise and in the duration of their effects. Post-traumatic stress disorder or recovered memory syndrome, for example, can be expressed in the widest variety of symptoms, which may arise long after the traumatic events believed to have triggered them. There is also a widespread conviction that these may continue indefinitely as people are 'scarred for life' by past traumas. Today's sufferers from addictions or compulsions can never claim to have been cured; they live their lives 'one day at a time' in an on-going process of 'recovery'.

The depersonalised character of traditional diagnoses allowed the sufferer to objectify the condition as something 'out there', perhaps a somewhat forced abstraction, but one with some pragmatic value. By contrast, a diagnosis like 'chronic fatigue syndrome', or 'ME', is inescapably personal and subjective in character. Every sufferer exhibits a different range of symptoms, and there is no way of objectively confirming or monitoring the course of the illness (Wessely 1998). The net effect of the dramatic expansion in the range of psychiatric diagnosis is that, instead of conferring strength on the patient, bestowing any such label is more likely to intensify and prolong incapacity. The proliferation of diagnoses and the tendency to apply them to ever wider sections of the population reflects a profound demoralisation of society and a deep crisis of subjectivity. To illustrate these trends, let's look at one example – addiction.

Hooked on addiction

Over the past decade a sense of heightened individual vulnerability in society has fostered a climate in which people are more and more inclined to attribute responsibility for their behaviour to someone – or something – outside themselves. Thus adults attribute their difficulties in relationships to emotional traumas inflicted on them in early childhood by their parents, students blame their teachers for their poor performance in exams, everybody seeks compensation from somebody else for their misfortunes. In this climate, the concept of addiction, that 'a substance or activity can produce a compulsion to act that is beyond the individual's self control' has a powerful resonance (Peele 1985: xi). As sociologist Frank Furedi puts it, 'the ideal of the self-determining individual has given way to a more diminished interpretation of subjectivity and the pathology of addiction provides a new standard for determining behaviour' (Furedi, forthcoming).

Alcoholism provides the model of a disease defined by uncontrollable behaviour which can readily be adapted to other activities deemed to be compulsive. The American critic of addiction Stanton Peele observes that 'there are an awful lot of things that people do that they know they shouldn't or that they regret doing more of than they want to'. However, 'once this pattern has been defined as a disease, almost anything can be treated as a medical problem' (Peele 1995: 117). Whereas the struggle to medicalise alcoholism raged for more than a century, the extension of the disease model of addiction, first from alcohol to heroin and tobacco, and then to gambling, shopping and sex has taken place over only a few years.

Though there were attempts to advance a disease theory of alcoholism from the end of the eighteenth century, the medical model made little headway against the powerful forces of religion and temperance until after the Second World War (Murphy 1996). During this period the conception of excessive drinking as a moral problem, as a vice demanding punishment, remained ascendant over the notion of alcoholism as a disease requiring treatment. It was not until the 1950s and 1960s, as the influence of religion declined and that of medicine increased, that the 'disease concept of alcoholism' gradually gained acceptance (Jellinek 1960). In 1977 the World Health Organisation adopted the term 'alcohol dependence syndrome', reflecting the new emphasis on 'chemical dependency' as the underlying pathology. By the 1980s, programmes of 'detoxification' and 'rehabilitation' under the control of the medical and psychiatric professions became the established forms of treating the problems of alcoholism.

The establishment of medical jurisdiction over opiate, specifically heroin, addiction was more straightforward, for a number of reasons (Berridge 1999). First, until the 1960s, it was a marginal problem: according to one account, 'there were so few heroin addicts in Britain that nearly all of them were known personally to the Home Office Drugs Branch Inspectorate' (BMA 1997: 7). Second, most of these were 'anxious middle aged professional people' (indeed many were doctors or nurses) who were not regarded as a threat to society. Third, heroin, a synthetic opiate first introduced (for its non-addictive qualities!) in 1895, was a prescription drug, with a 'medical' means of administration, the hypodermic syringe. In 1926 the Rolleston Report firmly defined heroin addiction as a disease and inaugurated the 'British system' of medical supervision. In the USA a more prohibitionist approach continued to criminalise heroin, with the effect, as in the sphere of alcohol, of encouraging illicit supply networks (Berridge 1979).

It was not until the 1970s and 1980s, that heroin abuse became identified as a significant social problem, now associated with an 'underclass' of alienated and marginalised youth. This resulted in some tension between the medical profession and the criminal justice system as the civil authorities insisted on tighter methods of regulation, as well as imposing harsher penalties on users and dealers. As we have seen, the penal and medical approaches subsequently converged in the extensive methadone maintenance programmes of the 1990s. The drug which has played a key role in the recent popularisation of the concept of addiction is one which was not considered addictive at all before the 1980s – tobacco.

Nicotine: from bad habit to chemical dependency

> Most smokers do not continue to smoke out of choice, but because they are addicted to nicotine.
>
> (RCP 2000: xiv)

This statement in the latest edition of the report by the Royal College of Physicians that launched the public campaign against smoking in the early 1960s reflects a significant shift in the war against tobacco and a confirmation of the current status of the concept of addiction. Whereas earlier editions had characterised smoking as a bad habit, the February 2000 version, bluntly titled *Nicotine Addiction in Britain*, claims that smokers are in the grip of a chemical dependency. According to the RCP report, its recognition of the addictive character of nicotine was a result of new researches in psychopharmacology, involving biochemical and behavioural studies in animals in humans. It seems probable that a greater influence was the growing popularity of notions of addiction in society generally. The RCP report conducted a detailed comparison of nicotine with heroin, cocaine, alcohol, caffeine, and concluded that nicotine was a 'highly addictive drug', by some criteria more so than some of these notorious drugs of abuse (RCP 2000: 100). Though this comparison was designed to reinforce the pernicious character of nicotine, it also implicitly undermined the wider concept of addiction: after all, if millions of people have managed to quit smoking and overcome the demon nicotine, perhaps the grip of heroin and cocaine is not quite the overwhelming compulsion it is often made out to be.

For the anti-smoking campaign, labelling nicotine as addictive is crucial to its challenge to the tobacco industry's insistence on 'consumer sovereignty', on the freedom of the individual to choose whether or not to buy cigarettes. As the RCP put it, 'if smoking and nicotine are addictive, the argument that the individual adult consumer has the right to choose to purchase and use tobacco products, and that the tobacco industry has the right to continue to supply them, is difficult to sustain' (RCP 2000: 101). If the smoker is the victim of a chemical dependency, and cigarettes are delivery systems for this chemical, then the government should regulate the supply and distribution of cigarettes as it would any other dangerous drug. Though the anti-smoking lobby plays up its offensive against the tobacco industry (whose executives are now despised and demonised as though they were war criminals or child abusers) its real threat is to the status of the individual and to civil liberties. If people who smoke – more than a quarter of the adult population – are defined as being in a state of drug addiction and are considered as a result to be incapable of making rational decisions, then the state is justified in taking ever greater control over their behaviour.

The dominant theme in the earlier medical literature was that cigarette smoking was merely a bad habit. That this habit could be broken by an effort of will was confirmed by the rapid response of an informed public to the revelations of the link between cigarettes and lung cancer. As we saw in Chapter 3, publicity about the dangers of smoking following the RCP's 1962 report led to a steady decline in levels of smoking. In a chapter devoted to 'the smoking habit', the second edition of the RCP report acknowledged discussion of 'pharmacological dependence' on nicotine (RCP 1971: 112) Though it suggested that this matter required further research, its general tone was dismissive: 'evidence that the difficulty that many smokers find in giving up the habit is due to habituation to nicotine is scanty' (RCP 1971: 41).

In the course of the 1960s and 1970s a wide range of programmes, using everything from behavioural and psychodynamic therapies to hypnotism and acupuncture, were established in the effort to encourage people to quit smoking. A review of these programmes in the USA in 1982 drew gloomy conclusions:

1   No one cessation technique or approach is clearly superior to any other;
2   Most people who join cessation programmes do not quit smoking;
3   Of those who do quit, most do not remain off cigarettes for any substantial period of time.

(Syme, Alcalay 1982)

Given the evident difficulty experienced by some in breaking the nicotine habit, and in the wider context of concern about 'drug dependency', the concept of nicotine addiction attracted increasing interest (Berridge 1998).

In the course of the 1980s, the recognition of nicotine addiction allowed for the convergence of different forms of dependence in the concept of 'substance abuse', or in the less judgemental term increasingly favoured in medical circles, 'substance misuse'. This provided a useful umbrella to cover not only alcohol, heroin and nicotine, but other illicit 'substances' – such as cannabis, solvents, cocaine/crack, amphetamines, LSD and ecstasy, and others – which were in widespread use, but for which the evidence of 'dependency' was weak.

If smokers were addicted to nicotine, then they needed treatment. Indeed they needed 'nicotine replacement therapy', a formulation paying richly ironic homage to the use of 'hormone replacement therapy' in post-menopausal women. A blood nicotine assay had become available for research purposes and nicotine chewing gum came on the market. In 1988 the US Surgeon-General's report gave official approval to nicotine addiction as a condition requiring appropriate medical treatment (Berridge 1998).

In Britain, however, some medical resistance to the concept of 'nicotine replacement therapy' was reflected in the decision not to make it available on prescription, either in the form of chewing gum or the more 'medical' skin patches. It was not until 1998 that an editorial in the *BMJ* called for 'nicotine replacement therapy for a healthier nation' – and proposed that it should be made available on prescription (Smeeth, Fowler 1998). This demand was issued with the full authority of a Cochrane Library 'systematic review' of 47 trials involving more than 23,000 patients, claiming to demonstrate its efficacy (Silagy *et al.* 1998). However, patients in these trials were only followed up for 6–12 months, so whether the effect is sustained remains unknown – as does whether this approach would also be effective when extended to a wider, and inevitably less motivated population. Nevertheless the nicotine replacement bandwagon was on the roll, and, following the RCP's enthusiastic endorsement, it seems set to allow the further medicalisation of individual behaviour.

Co-dependency

The key factor in enabling the concept of addiction to extend beyond dependence on chemical substances was the emergence in the USA of the 'co-dependency' movement. The roots of this movement, the subject of a penetrating study by John Steadman Rice, lie in the 'Twelve Step' recovery programme popularised by Alcoholics Anonymous (founded in Ohio in 1935, AA became widely established in the USA and internationally in the post-war period) (Steadman Rice 1998). Though groups concerned with the special problems of the spouses and families of alcoholics had long run in parallel with the mainstream AA meetings, in the 1980s there was a dramatic proliferation of such groups. They now rapidly expanded to include 'survivors' of other forms of victimisation (domestic violence, sexual abuse) and victims of other forms of addiction, such as gambling, shopping, sex. The central claim of this movement was that 'co-dependency' was a disease, an addiction, characterised by dependence on a pathological relationship with another person, a substance, or any 'processes external to the individual' (Steadman Rice 1998).

Co-dependents are believed to experience 'a pattern of painful dependence on compulsive behaviours and on approval from others in an attempt to find safety, self worth and identity'. As Steadman Rice observes, this is a concept of 'virtually limitless applicability' and it was not surprising to find it extending to cover, not only familiar bad habits, but even fads about novelties such as the internet, mobile phones and the National Lottery (all of which were linked with media scare stories about new forms of addiction in the late 1990s). The inevitable result was inflated estimates of the numbers of victims of various addictions: one (US) estimate reckoned that co-dependency afflicted 'approximately 96 per cent of the population' (Steadman Rice 1998) Lest this be thought to be a preoccupation peculiar to Americans, the British advocacy group Action on Addiction claims that 'almost every one of us has either experienced some form of addiction or knows someone who has' (AOA 1997). With typically British modesty it settles for the assertion that 'in fact, one in three adults suffer from some form of addiction'.

While co-dependency expanded the concept of addiction to cover diverse personal and social problems, there was also a surge in the popularity of biological theories of addiction. Developments in genetics (not only a 'gene for alcoholism', but also a 'promiscuity gene'), advances in the study of neurotransmitters (endorphins, serotonin, dopamine) and the speculations of evolutionary psychologists were all recruited to explain the remarkable grip of compulsions and addictions on individuals in modern society (James 1997). The crude biological determinism apparent in such attempts to establish a direct link of causality that extends from embryonic DNA, through the structure and function of the brain to the individual personality and social behaviour reflects the profoundly fatalistic outlook that underlies the concept of addiction. If human behaviour is 'hard wired' into our genes and hormones, then the scope for individual autonomy and self-control is drastically curtailed. The culture of addiction is assiduously promoted by the therapeutic entrepreneurs of the worlds of counselling and therapy and by the cults of self-help, personal growth and victim support.

Bookshop shelves are heaving with manuals of pop psychology and numerous websites provide similar wisdom in an easily accessible form for the internet generation. Both often provide handy checklists against which readers can assess whether they qualify for the diagnosis of co-dependency (the answer, of course, is yes). Two young men have come into the surgery, having completed one such checklist confirming the diagnosis of the adult form of attention deficit hyperactivity disorder. Indeed both had poor records at school, difficulties in maintaining jobs and relationships, problems with the law: how about some Ritalin (the amphetamine-type drug recommended for ADHD)? The propaganda of addiction finds a ready resonance in a society in which people are all too ready to accept a medical label for their difficulties.

The inflation of addiction is a morbid social symptom. It encourages people to regard themselves as passive victims of external forces, of demonised 'substances' or 'toxic' relationships, even of their own biology. The widespread acceptance of this outlook is all the more remarkable if you consider the extent to which it contradicts most people's experience. As Peele writes, 'people regularly quit smoking, cut back drinking, lose weight, improve their health, create healthy love relationships, raise strong and happy children and contribute to communities and combat wrong – all without expert intervention' (Peele 1995: 29). As I indicated above, I would also add 'get off drugs'. I wonder whether expert intervention is in fact often counterproductive. This is most clearly apparent in relation to methadone maintenance where the goal of abstinence is replaced with that of indefinite dependence. But there is also a marked tendency for vulnerable people to develop an ongoing dependence on therapy, which is as likely to confirm their inadequacy as it is to enable them to overcome it.

Counselling and Prozac

Doctors of all sorts, notably psychiatrists and GPs, have helped to encourage the inflation of addiction and other psychological disorders and the demand for medical or psychological treatment that follows from it. Experts are continually advising us of the need to identify problem drinkers and others with 'substance abuse' problems so that they can be offered appropriate treatment. In 1992 the *Health of the Nation* white paper identified mental health as a key area and, for the first time, set targets on reducing the suicide rate. The neglect of any means of achieving this (or indeed its other targets) meant that this policy had little consequence, but this defect was remedied when the New Labour government after 1997 also established a target. It also sponsored a 'Defeat Depression' campaign, which sought to encourage GPs to increase their diagnosis of depression, in the hope that this would facilitate treatment and thus reduce the suicide rate. Treatments on offer in the surgery fall into two broad categories: counselling and medication.

A *BMJ* editorial in 1993 noted that, even though 'many attempts to evaluate its effectiveness have shown little or no benefit', counselling had rapidly become established in general practice in Britain (Pringle, Laverty 1993). The authors noted that 'as well as its general indications in anxiety and depression, and problems with relationships', counselling had been advocated for 'smoking cessation, modification of diet, alcohol misuse, postnatal depression, addiction to tranquillisers, and high risk sexual behaviour'. The government-imposed GP contract in 1990 had encouraged the provision of counselling in general practice by agreeing to reimburse up to 70 per cent of the cost. The later growth of fund-holding practices gave a further boost to the employment of counsellors in the surgery.

The theme of Pringle and Laverty's editorial was 'reasons for caution' about the explosion of counselling in general practice, given the lack of evidence of effectiveness and uncertainties about confidentiality, qualifications and accreditation. There was a generally negative response to their editorial, and particularly to their suggestion that 'the main reason for GPs' enthusiasm for counselling may well be a desire to reduce contact with and responsibility for a very demanding group of patients'. One critic insisted that GPs 'were not just avoiding "heartsink" patients, as the editorial suggests, but recognised the mutual benefit of bringing new skills and knowledge into the practice and extending the range of options within the primary care team' (Jewell 1993). Counselling was one of those initiatives whose value was considered self-evident. Attempts to investigate its effectiveness were all very well, but should not be allowed to delay its implementation.

The provision of counselling in GPs' surgeries was a radical departure with a number of significant features, not the least of which was the fact that it generally passed without much comment. It indicated that GPs were prepared to provide treatment, within the framework of the primary health care team, for a range of personal problems not previously considered to fall within the sphere of medical practice. Furthermore they were prepared to refer their own patients to unregistered practitioners in a way which, a few years earlier, would have led to a summons to appear before the General Medical Council. As GP Myles Harris, one of the few critics of this trend, pointed out, 'the idea of the medical register was to protect the public against untested therapies and counselling has no substantial agreed body of scientific evidence to back its claims' (Harris 1994: 24). Harris was concerned that doctors were turning their backs on their traditions of scientific medicine and 'in allowing counsellors into the NHS we may be deserting medicine for magic'.

The fact that the government agreed to subsidise these counselling services indicated that it was 'ready to treat ordinary human difficulties as illnesses' (Harris 1994: 6). Yet this also carried the danger of allowing the state, through the agency of counsellors, to define 'what is "normal" in everyday behaviour'. The fact that coun-selling was already mandatory for HIV testing revealed the tendency towards compulsion that is often closely linked to the idea of normality. Harris rightly alerted GPs to the authoritarian implications of what was generally regarded as a beneficent policy.

The alternative to counselling was drugs – and the drug of the 1990s was Prozac. In the past doctors had been drawn into treating unhappiness with barbiturates (such as Seconal and Nembutal), in the 1950s and 1960s, and with benzodiazepines (such as Valium and Librium) in the 1960s and 1970s. Drugs from both groups had been used on a large scale, causing serious problems of overdose and long-term dependence. The development of tricyclic antidepressants (Imipramine and Amitriptyline) in the 1960s had improved the treatment of depression, but the high incidence of side-effects limited their use. Numerous attempts to produce similar drugs without causing a dry mouth, blurred vision, constipation and other adverse reactions proved disappointing. 'This was the stage onto which Prozac walked: thirty years of stasis', wrote Peter Kramer in his classic account (Kramer 1994: 60). Prozac, the trade name for Fluoxetine, is the best known of the 'selective serotonin reuptake inhibitors', which first appeared in the late 1980s. After a quiet start, Prozac featured in *Newsweek* magazine in 1990 and a 'celebrity career' took off. By the end of the year 650,000 prescriptions for it were being issued every month in the USA and by 1993, five years after its release, eight million people had taken it, half of them abroad. It appears that this group of drugs is effective in relieving depression in some people and that fewer patients get side-effects while taking them. They are fairly safe in overdose and do not seem to cause dependency.

The question set by Prozac in the context of the inflation of psychological illness is – what proportion of the population should be on it? As Kramer observed, 'psychiatric diagnosis had already been subject to a sort of "diagnostic bracket creep" – the expansion of categories to match the scope of relevant medications' (Kramer 1994: 15). He emphasised that 'how large a sphere of human problems we choose to define as medical is an important social decision'. For Oliver James, the answer was simple: shortly before the 1997 general election he advised Jack Straw, who subsequently became home secretary, that the twenty million people he considered to be in need of intervention should all receive Prozac. He reported that Straw was 'mildly amused at such a mechanistic formulation' though this did not discourage James from his conviction that this was 'a useful way of thinking about the problems he faces in his job' (James 1997: 307).

Meanwhile, down in the surgery, the trend towards what Kramer calls the 'medicalisation of personality' is proceeding apace. The result is not only an enormously increased workload, but the inevitability of failing to meet the expectations raised by the indiscriminate application of medical labels to diverse forms of existential distress. Prozac may become a little helper to mother and the rest of the family, but it will not provide a long-term solution to the problems of a diminished self. People may seek a 'detox' from the problems of life but, as everybody knows, it is not withdrawal that is difficult, but living an independent life.

7

THE PERSONAL IS THE MEDICAL

The widening scope of medical practice is not confined to the diagnosis and treatment of psychological disturbance. Doctors have become increasingly involved in the regulation of the more intimate and personal aspects of their patients' lives, seeking to influence their conduct of intimate relationships. Thus GPs are now exhorted to take an active interest in patients' sexual behaviour, to be alert to all possible manifestations of domestic violence and to promote parenting skills.

Different influences have pushed these concerns into the GP's surgery, moving with different dynamics over the past decade. The new discipline of 'sexual health' indicated the creation of a link between 'sex' and 'health', two formerly autonomous, if not antagonistic, spheres of human endeavour. (In practice, the links assiduously promoted by the Aids establishment were between sex and disease, pleasure and death.) As the Aids scare faltered in the early 1990s, activists turned to running training courses for GPs to encourage them to do more work in the field of sexual health. A series of public controversies around issues of child protection in the 1980s led to the formulation of policies requiring closer involvement of GPs in issues of child protection. The growing influence of feminism in public life, catalysed by the election of the New Labour government in Britain in 1997, brought the crusade against domestic violence into the surgery, with a plethora of guidelines and recommendations in the late 1990s. The new government also gave a priority to public health and to issues of 'inequalities' in health and welfare and 'social exclusion'. These policies did not involve any redistribution of resources to the poor (the anathematised tradition of Old Labour); in practice, they meant more intensive measures to push people into the labour market and schemes to foster healthy lifestyles and parenting skills – which is where GPs come in.

Initiatives in all these areas are regarded as being at the cutting edge of progressive general practice and are likely to receive generous financial support from government and voluntary agencies. Any suggestion that this extension of professional inter-vention into the personal sphere, and the implicit shifting of the boundary between the public and the private, might have adverse consequences for the autonomy of the individual and the stability of the family, is dismissed as yet another voice of the forces of conservatism trying to hold back the tide of progress. Let's look more closely at the role of the GP in the bedroom, the living room and the nursery.

Sex in the surgery

Shortly before the millennium, we were bombarded at the health centre with invitations to attend a 'sexuality training day' on the subject of 'sex in primary care'. I requested details of the agenda which promised 'an opportunity to discuss [my] experience of sexual history taking, explore associated issues and develop and enhance [my] skills and confidence to discuss sex with a diverse range of patients'. Highlights of a day featuring games and role play included an 'orgasm exercise': 'pairs to practice communications skills to talk about experience of or understanding of an orgasm'. Another exercise tackled 'sexual language': 'small groups to brainstorm words for Male and Female sexual organs and homosexual/homosexuality'. The course included 'a nice lunch and all course materials'(!).

My first response was to regard this course as rather silly and self-indulgent, as yet another example of the 'dumbing down' of postgraduate education. But, if we ask the question – how is a sexuality training day for GPs supposed to relate to their work with patients? – we raise a deeper problem. It is clear that the aim of the course is to overcome doctors' own inhibitions in talking about sex so that they can in turn break through their patients' reserve in these matters. Challenging doctors' personal reticence is the key to opening up the intimate areas of ordinary people's lives to professional scrutiny and interference.

The 'Sex and the GP' conference, one of many such training initiatives, is part of a wider campaign to encourage GPs to play a more interventionist role in their patients' sexual health. In 1995, for example, the BMA Foundation for Aids sent a complimentary copy of *Sexual health promotion in general practice* (retail price £15) to every GP in London (Curtis *et al.* 1995). 'What's so special about this book?' asked an effusive accompanying letter. '*This book is unique.* It is the only book on sexual health promotion which has been written and presented in an attractive, readable format *specifically* for busy doctors, nurses and other staff working in general practice.' This meant that it was largely written in bullet points, reflecting its authors' judgement that professionals working in primary health care lack the intellectual capacity to read prose.

The main justification offered for this well-resourced drive to recruit GPs to the safe sex crusade was that it was part of the campaign to reduce the incidence of HIV and other sexually transmitted diseases. This did not make much sense as both HIV and STDs are fairly uncommon in general practice and also because there is a flourishing network of clinics already dealing with these problems. So why target general practice? The free sexual health handbook provides a long list of the 'advantages' of general practice as 'a setting for promoting sexual health', of which the first three are:

- Reaches large numbers of people on a one-to-one basis
- Relationship with patient already exists
- Opportunities to discuss sexual health arise during relevant consultations, for example, for smears or contraception.

The importance of general practice is that it provides access to the mass of the population through an individual who has a relationship with people that reaches deep into their personal, private space.

The central concern of sexual health promotion is not to prevent disease but to preach a new form of sexual morality. The distinctive feature of this moral code is that it explicitly disclaims being a moral code. Yet the new framework simply replaces 'good' with 'safe' and 'evil' with 'unsafe' and proceeds to construct a code as dogmatic and authoritarian as any to be found in the Bible or the Koran. *Sexual health promotion in general practice* provides a table of around 30 forms of sexual activity which are classified, fairly arbitrarily, as 'safe/low risk; possibly safe/medium risk; unsafe/high risk'. Like scholars of the Talmud, the rabbinate of the sexual health establishment finds fruitful employment in tutoring the faithful in the subtleties of the classification and in offering endless interpretations and reinterpretations of the sacred text. Those who stray from the path of righteousness – such as the HIV positive woman discovered in the summer of 1999 to be breastfeeding her baby (a behaviour of indeterminate risk) – are likely to find themselves smitten with the full force of the law, not to mention the wrath of the media.

It is interesting to contrast the process of medicalisation of sex that is taking place today with that in the late nineteenth century. One of the insights of the French philosopher Michel Foucault was that the apparent liberalisation associated with the sexual reformers of the late Victorian period was illusory. By identifying and classifying diverse forms of sexual experience, they merely replaced a traditional mode of moral regulation with a modern, rational, professionally-mediated form of surveillance and control (Foucault 1979). The 'repeal of reticence' led to the displacement of the priest by the doctor, whose supervision was more thorough.

Yet the resulting 'revolution in manners and morals' remained largely confined to the elite of society, in Britain scarcely extending beyond the Bloomsbury set. The distinctive feature of the current phase of medicalisation is that it reaches out to the whole of society and penetrates more deeply into the individual personality. When Foucault commented on the replacement of 'silence' with 'volubility' about sex in the 1890s, he can scarcely have anticipated the combined effect of contemporary television discussions about sex and an encounter with a family GP after a 'sexuality training day'. Reticence may be in shreds, but this has been achieved at the cost of the intrusion of the doctor into the bedroom and the transformation of the doctor's surgery into a confessional.

Domestic violence

There has been some controversy among medical authorities concerned with the problem of domestic violence about whether or not all patients should be asked, as a matter of routine, whether they are currently experiencing any form of assault from their partner (BMA 1998). If women are asked about domestic violence only if they come in with a black eye, then many instances of abuse, which may leave less conspicuous but no less profound injuries, may go unrecorded. If, on the other hand, all women are asked routinely, then this reduces the stigma surrounding the whole issue and makes it easier for them to disclose the nature and extent of their victimhood. Such direct questioning may, however, upset some women who only came to see their doctor with a sore throat or a verruca.

Noting that US guidelines now recommend direct questioning as a routine, irrespective of the complaint that has brought the patient to the doctor, the authors of a BMA report on domestic violence fear that traditional reserve still inhibits such an approach in Britain (BMA 1998). Still, they are clearly hopeful that a growing awareness of domestic violence will make routine questioning about intimate aspects of women's private lives more widely acceptable.

Domestic violence suddenly became a major preoccupation of the health establishment in the late 1990s. In addition to the BMA book, the Royal College of Obstetrics and Gynaecology and the Royal College of Midwives both issued statements on the subject (Bewley et al. 1997; Royal College of Midwives 1997). The Chief Medical Officer highlighted domestic violence in his 1996 report and in 1999 the Royal College of General Practioners circulated guidelines on 'the GP's role' (DoH 1997; Heath 1999). All these publications sought to raise awareness of domestic violence among health professionals and to encourage a more interventionist, pro-active approach to the problem.

Discussing this matter with my GP colleagues, who are mainly women, I inquired whether they had noticed a recent upsurge in domestic violence. But no; like me, they had certainly encountered the occasional case, but thought it not a very common problem and had not noted any particular increase. Of course, our low recognition of domestic violence may be a result of our limited conception of the problem, which has been radically redefined by campaigners. Following current conventions, the BMA distinguishes three types of domestic violence: physical, sexual and psychological. The latter category includes criticism, verbal abuse and 'being forced to do menial/trivial tasks' as well as humiliation and degradation, extreme jealousy/possessiveness and 'being made to think they are going mad'. Using this definition the final estimate of prevalence is that 'one in four women will experience domestic violence at some time in their lives'. The only surprise is that it is not closer to 100 per cent.

The 'one in four' statistic is repeated in all the recent reports and it echoes around any lecture theatre or conference hall in which domestic violence is discussed. It is worth examining one of the key sources of this figure, which is referenced in all current handbooks and guidelines – a major survey of domestic violence in North London, conducted under the aegis of Middlesex University and Islington Council (Mooney 1993). The study adopted a definition of domestic violence, similar to that of the BMA, as conduct including 'mental cruelty, threats, sexual abuse, physical violence and any other form of controlling behaviour' (Mooney 1993: 8). The team of researchers conducting the interviews were 'all chosen for their understanding of and commitment to the problem of domestic violence' and given 'intensive training' (Mooney 1993: 10). The first stage of the study took the form of an interview and the completion of a questionnaire, conducted with the researcher and the subject alone together. This aimed to clarify the subject's perception of what constituted domestic violence. The next stage involved the subject completing a more extensive questionnaire in private; in the final stage women who had experienced violence had a further 'in depth' interview.

The key encounter here is the first stage interview between a researcher chosen for her 'commitment to the problem of domestic violence' and the subject, who has generously given up her time and is keen to be helpful to a project she knows to be concerned about the issue of domestic violence. The fact that they are alone protects the subject from external influences (an understandable precaution if the interview is in the subject's home), but it inevitably also maximises the influence of the researcher. The result is clearly more of a tutorial than an investigation: it is not surprising that, as they talk over different 'vignettes of conflict situations' the subject's definition of domestic violence tends to expand to correspond with that of the investigator. It is also not surprising that this approach yields results which suggest levels of domestic violence vastly greater than those recorded in conventional crime surveys, which include questions about domestic violence in wider questionnaires (and report rates of between 2 and 4 per cent).While Mooney seeks to explain this difference by the greater accuracy of her findings, the real explanation lies in her methodology.

Mooney notes with approval the subjects' 'acceptance of a broad definition of domestic violence'. She concludes that 'clearly ... women's prioritisation of this range of experience under the rubric of domestic violence would suggest a demand for a wide range of agency intervention' (Mooney 1993: 23). What is clear from this exercise is that Mooney and her team, motivated by a 'commitment to the problem of domestic violence' and keen to promote 'a wide range of intervention' to deal with it, have successfully recruited their research subjects to their definition of the problem and to their strategy for dealing with it.

Though the BMA report concedes that much of the research on which its conclusions are based is 'not of high quality', this does not deter it from recycling spurious statistics. Thus, for example, it quotes a major survey of GPs in Canada which revealed that 'almost all believed that they are missing cases of abuse and just over half of respondents estimated that they are missing 30% or more cases' (BMA, 1998: 37). Such GPs, who can estimate the percentage of an unknown quantity, are wasted in general practice (though they might find a successful career in epidemiology).

'What are we supposed to do about it?' was the rather weary chorus from my colleagues when I raised their awareness of the campaign to raise their awareness about domestic violence. One of the more interesting findings of the North London survey was a high level of satisfaction with their GPs among women who had disclosed domestic violence to them (Mooney 1993: 54). These obviously rather old-fashioned doctors were handicapped by the fact that they had had 'no access to domestic violence awareness training'. Nevertheless, they had been sympathetic, providing a listening ear and helpful reports in relation to court cases and housing problems (though there was some suggestion that, more recently, they appeared to have less time to devote to these problems). These GPs clearly need some training in the more interventionist approach, which recommends immediate and long-term responses.

The immediate response is a series of measures that encourage the victim towards involving other agencies, most importantly the police and the courts. There is a general approval of the fact that the police have adopted a much more interventionist approach, setting up domestic violence units and being ready to enforce court orders against violent spouses or partners. It is striking, however, that in this era of evidence-based practice, no evidence is adduced that the intervention of the police and the criminal justice system provides effective protection for women. The tragic case of Vandana Patel, fatally stabbed by her husband inside the domestic violence unit of our local police station in Stoke Newington in 1991, indicates that the police cannot guarantee women's security. One of the few critics of the feminist enthusiasm for a more coercive approach to domestic violence – American academic Jean Bethke Elshtain – notes that 'scant attention gets paid to the danger that enhancing police prerogatives to intervene may lead to abuse of the society's least powerful' (Elshtain, 1998: 174).

The long-term consequence of GPs adopting a more pro-active approach to domestic violence is more insidious. It means opening up the personal realm of family life and relationships to professional interference on an unprecedented scale. The BMA report comments that the doctor is in a particularly good position to intervene, because he or she does 'not necessarily need to prove the existence of domestic violence ... but instead needs to identify and acknowledge that domestic violence is occurring' (BMA 1998: 45). The doctor's suspicion of violence is thus deemed to justify unleashing a comprehensive programme of intervention, possibly involving a wide range of local authority and voluntary organisations, as well as other health professionals.

A popular model is the Domestic Abuse Intervention Project in Duluth, Minnesota, USA. This seeks through multi-agency working to transform a range of violent behaviour into non-violent or egalitarian behaviour, showing respect and trust, giving support, being honest and accountable, fairly negotiating, taking shared responsiblity, having economic partnership and responsible parenting. Whether or not this approach is effective in terms of deterring domestic violence, it carries the heavy cost of opening up the private sphere to public scrutiny and regulation in a way that is characteristic of authoritarian societies. Such an intrusion into the intimate life of the individual can only be profoundly damaging both for the individual and for society.

Again Elshtain is alert to the oppressive consequences of domestic violence programmes:

> Mandated counselling, even behavioural conditioning of violent men, coupled with compulsory punishment, are common as part of the panoply of interim proposals, along with a refusal to think about potential abuses inherent in extending therapeutic powers and responsibilities to the state as part of its policing function.
>
> (Elshstain, 1998: 174)

She warns of the danger that the crusade against domestic violence may result in a world of 'total scrutiny, total accountability, and instant justice' in which 'the social space for difference, indifference, dissent, and refusal is squeezed out' (Elshtain 1998: 175).

In the Canadian survey cited above, of the 21 reasons given by GPs for not identifying more cases of domestic violence, the two *least* common, were 'it is not a medical matter' and it's 'none of my business'. Though these may be the convictions of a minority, they point the way forward to a form of medical practice that treats illness rather than regulating behaviour and puts the autonomy of the individual and the privacy of personal life before the imperatives of political correctness.

The dangers of family support

The key event in catalysing the transformation of general practice into an interventionist agency of social control was the election of the New Labour government in May 1997. A central theme of New Labour policy is the need for 'joined-up solutions' to 'joined-up problems'. The government's central preoccupation is with the fragmentation of society, most conspicuously expressed in the priority it gives to dealing with 'social exclusion'. In response to the perceived problems of social disintegration it is keen to promote any manifestation of collectivity and to encourage any form of collaboration among agencies and professionals that might help to restore community and cohesion. The focus of the government's public health programme – especially its flagship 'health action zones' – is on promoting local networks, inter-agency working, flexibility in professional roles. The idea is to take advantage of the popularity of primary health care services (GPs, district nurses, midwives, etc.) to restore the bonds of neighbourhood and community that have been severely eroded by the social and political trends of the past decade. Given the fact that doctors and nurses have managed to retain much higher levels of popular approval than social workers and other professionals, it is not surprising to find that the GP surgery has been identified as a suitable focus for the strategy of promoting local networks. A *Guardian/ICM* poll in January 2000 asked people to grade various professionals (on a scale of 1–10) according to how they were 'respected by people in general': doctors came in at 8.4, exceeded only by nurses (8.5). Cabinet ministers and MPs tied at 5.5 (18 January). At a time when other agencies – notably social services – are held in low regard, they appear to have devised a strategy of reorganising around primary health care, in the hope that this will increase their public acceptability.

The development of initiatives in the sphere of primary care that involve collaboration with social workers, sometimes in voluntary organisations, around 'family support' is one consequence of the New Labour approach to social problems. One such scheme – the WellFamily Project – was piloted in Hackney and a number of other areas in the late 1990s and has been widely recommended as a model for the primary care intervention in the family (Layzell, Graffy 1998; Goodhart et al. 1999). The project was developed by GPs working in collaboration with the Family Welfare Association, a voluntary organisation with roots in Victorian philanthropy. The FWA provided a 'family support coordinator', who was qualified as a health visitor and had undergone further training in 'family therapy, solution-focused counselling and welfare rights'. Individuals or families, considered to be in need of psychological, emotional or practical support were referred by the GPs in a group practice and were seen by the family support worker in the surgery. Some were seen only once and offered information and advice or referral to another agency. Others received brief counselling over several sessions (between two and five). Around 20 per cent required longer-term support.

'At a time when social services are overburdened in Britain', observes Clare Goodhart, the GP heading the project, 'family support in general practice offers one way to fill the gap' (Goodhart et al. 1999). Many GPs might think that their surgeries were as overburdened as the social services and wonder whether it was their job to 'fill the gap' resulting from the inadequacy of local authority social care provision. However, initial reports suggested a high level of satisfaction with this project for everybody involved. For the GPs, the family support worker provided a point of referral for patients whose social or emotional difficulties were expressed in inappropriate requests for medical treatments. Patients liked being referred to a social worker within the surgery; the service was in a familiar and easily accessible place and, a point made repeatedly in the reports, it did not carry the stigma associated with local authority social services.

It is understandable that many of our patients, who are experiencing great difficulties in their lives, should welcome extra support from any direction. Yet, as the evaluation of the WellFamily project makes clear, 'family support' is not an entirely benign concept. The report indicates that, though there is no consensus over the definition of 'family support', there has been considerable debate about the relationship between this concept and that of 'child protection' and about the 'appropriate balance between the two' (Layzell, Graffy 1998: 6–7). The authors appear to maintain a distinction between intervention where the primary concern is the safety of the children ('protection') and 'preventative or early intervention strategies' ('support'). In other words support is being offered to families by the WellFamily Project as part of a strategy to prevent child abuse. The vigorously 'pro-active' character of the project (the support worker chases up clients by telephone or letter if they do not turn up for appointments) is consistent with this preventive approach (and distinguishes it from other parenting projects which have high default rates). But have patients given their informed consent to this form of intervention recommended by their GP and carried out in the surgery?

Project leaders emphasise the 'independent' and 'non-statutory' character of the 'family support coordinator' as a key to her acceptability and to the non-stigmatising character of the service (Goodhart *et al.* 1999). But, in relation to child protection, this independence is entirely notional: under the terms of the Children Act and the 'Working Together' guidelines, workers in primary health care as well as in local authority social services have clear responsibilities to report instances of child abuse (Home Office 1991). The authors conclude that 'whether stigma might transfer to the WellFamily Project remains to be seen' but they are optimistic that 'since the worker is not responsible for statutory child protection work she is unlikely to generate the same fears'. This confusion is unlikely to survive the first child protection case that arises and the transfer of stigma, over time, is inevitable.

The government's sponsorship of a series of initiatives to promote the teaching of parenting skills – the SureStart programme, the National Family and Parenting Institute and numerous subsidised voluntary organisations – has been criticised as an intrusion on parental autonomy (Fitzpatrick 1999). The notion that doctors should encourage, if not directly sponsor, such programmes is now widely accepted. Yet it marks a dramatic reversal of what was traditionally regarded as good medical practice. In an essay first published in 1950, the famous child psychotherapist Donald Winnicott insisted that 'we must see that we never interfere with a home that is a going concern, not even for its own good' (Winnicott 1965: 132). He warned that 'doctors are especially liable to get in the way between mothers and infants, or parents and children, always with the best intentions, for the prevention of disease and the promotion of health'. Winnicott, famed for his sensitivity to children's mental states, was acutely aware that intruding between children and their parents, who are the most reliable guarantor of their interests, could have a destabilising effect. In a later essay, entitled 'Advising Parents', Winnicott amplified his views. 'All my professional life', he began, 'I have avoided giving advice', indicating that he aimed to discourage other doctors from doing so (Winnicott 1965: 114). He carefully distinguished the legitimate sphere of medical intervention – the treatment of disease – from giving 'advice about life', which was beyond their competence:

> Doctors and nurses [should] understand that they do not have to settle problems of living for their clients, men and women who are often more mature persons than the doctor or nurse who is advising.
>
> (Winnicott 1965: 115)

According to Winnicott, for a doctor to advise people about such problems was not only impertinent, but implicitly authoritarian.

While offering information and support to parents, expert intervention diminishes the value of parents' intimate experience of dealing with their own children. The intrusion of an external source of authority into the family undermines not only confidence but also accountability. Any third party intrusion between parents and children (Furedi 2000) is likely to weaken their own capacities to work through and resolve conflicts. Though motivated by a desire to provide help and support to families in need, parenting projects are likely to weaken parental authority still further. If GPs generally take on a wider role in family support and the promotion of parenting, they will be drawn into a more intrusive and authoritarian approach to their patients. The result will be damaging to doctor–patient relationships, and inevitably to professional status. The relatively high standing of general practice which makes it such an attractive base for New Labour's moral engineering projects is a wasting asset, one likely to be expended very rapidly if GPs assume the shabby mantle of social work. It is rather ironic that, after seeking to take over the management of the social as well as the medical problems of the neighbourhood, many GPs complain of high levels of stress (not to mention a growing inclination among their patients to assault them).

8

THE CRISIS OF MODERN
MEDICINE

Bad doctors should no more expect to be employed by the
health service than bad teachers should expect to be employed by the education service. ... They would be 'named
and shamed'.

(Health Minister Alan Milburn, *Guardian*,
19 November 1998)

The conviction in January 2000 of Manchester GP Harold Shipman
of the murder of 15 of his patients could not have come at a better
time for the medical establishment. Following the scandal of the
high death rates at the Bristol children's heart surgery unit
(culminating in disciplinary action against three doctors in June
1998), the Kent gynaecologist Rodney Ledward (struck off the
medical register in October 1998 for gross negligence), and
numerous less grievous cases of incompetence or corruption, the
Shipman case provided further impetus to the drive to tighten
administrative control over the medical profession (Abbasi 1999).

In the closing months of 1999, a flurry of documents indicated
the direction of measures for tougher action against rogue or
'under-performing' doctors and for closer regulation of the
profession as a whole. The GMC published its long-awaited plans
for the regular 'revalidation' of doctors based on an assessment of
their fitness to practise (Buckley 1999). The RCGP and the General
Practitioners Committee of the BMA jointly produced proposals on
how revalidation could be implemented in general practice (RCGP
October 1999, November 1999). Meanwhile the government's chief
medical officer, Liam Donaldson, issued a consultation paper on
'preventing, recognising and dealing with poor performance' among
doctors, proposing 'assessment and support centres' – immediately
dubbed 'boot camps' or 'sin bins' – for delinquent doctors (DoH

November 1999). These measures to strengthen the regulation of medical practice overlapped with the drive to implement new systems of quality control under the banner of 'clinical governance'. The two key agencies overseeing this process – the National Institute of Clinical Excellence (NICE) and the Commission for Health Improvement (CHI) – opened for business in the course of 1999.

The government now adopted a higher profile in pursuing the reform of medical practice. In his party conference speech in September 1999, prime minister Tony Blair condemned the 'forces of conservatism' – specifically referring to the BMA – that were holding back the government's modernising reforms (*The Times*, 29 September). In fact, the forces of conservatism in the medical profession – indeed any forces of opposition to the drive towards tighter regulation – were difficult to discern. By contrast to its vigorous campaign against the Conservative reforms of the early 1990s, the BMA's response to the New Labour initiatives was generally favourable. Indeed, the distinctive feature of the late 1990s reforms was that they were backed by powerful forces within the profession. Influential professional bodies like the GMC and the royal colleges were broadly in favour of the reforms (indeed, in substance, they had initiated them). Behind the appearance of a radical, modernising government courageously imposing change on a reactionary medical profession lay a different dynamic. In the course of the 1990s a growing sense of professional insecurity among doctors was expressed in the vogue for clinical audit, the drive to use the measurement of performance to improve standards, and in the demand for guidelines for clinical practice. Following the election of the New Labour government in May 1997, the internal aspiration to raise standards converged with the external imperative to modernise the NHS by strengthening managerial control and diminishing professional autonomy. Far from confronting entrenched 'forces of conservatism' in the medical profession, New Labour was able to enter a close alliance with a new medical elite that identified closely with its policies. By contrast with the powerful 'forces of modernisation' in the health service, voices of opposition were few, isolated and defensive.

To grasp the scale of the crisis of professional confidence that engulfed medicine in the 1990s, we need to trace its emergence over the preceding decades. In the 1960s and 1970s medicine faced criticisms from insiders and radicals; in the 1980s these were taken over and broadened by outsiders and conservatives; in the 1990s the profession turned on itself. Such was the ideological disorder of the post-modern world that this process of professional self-abasement could be presented – and largely accepted – as a movement of radical reform.

The epidemiological transition

> Medicine, like many other American institutions, suffered a stunning loss of confidence in the 1970s.
>
> (Starr 1982: 379)

Though there is a consensus that the medical profession throughout the Western world experienced a profound crisis in the 1970s, there is less agreement about the nature of the crisis and its causes. As Paul Starr's formulation implies, this crisis was not confined to medicine, suggesting that we need to explore the interaction between the specific difficulties encountered in medical practice in this period and wider developments in society. It appears that, after the spectacular advances of the post-war years, the pace of medical innovation began to slow and the emergence of new problems revealed that, for all its achievements and its promise, scientific medicine was not without its deficiencies and dangers. In the course of the 1960s these issues came under discussion within the medical world – but had little wider impact. It was the social, economic and political turmoil that began in the late 1960s and continued through the next decade that led to a wider challenge to the medical profession (and to other established institutions and sources of authority). This opened up the discussion of the problems facing modern medicine to a wider audience and amplified the insecurities of the profession.

The publication of *The Mirage of Health* by the American micro-biologist Rene Dubos in 1960 marked the beginning of the end of the golden age of post-war medicine (though like many books which anticipate emerging trends, its significance was recognised much more in retrospect than at the time). Dubos, who had himself played a distinguished role in the development of antibiotics, acknowl-edged that one of the key principles of scientific medicine – the doctrine of specific aetiology, which held that every disease had a particular cause (a doctrine dramatically vindicated by the germ theory of infectious disease) which could, at least potentially be treated – was reaching the limits of its usefulness. 'Few are the cases', he wrote, 'in which it has provided a complete account of the causation of disease' (Dubos, 1960: 87). Though the methods of scientific medicine had proved effective in dealing with some infectious diseases, 'despite frantic efforts, the causes of cancer, of arteriosclerosis, of mental disorders, and of the great medical problems of our time remain undiscovered'. While many still believed that solutions could be found 'by bringing the big guns of science to bear on the problems', Dubos argued that the 'search for *the* cause may be a hopeless pursuit because most of the disease states are the indirect outcome of a constellation of circumstances rather than the direct result of single determinant factors'.

Dubos contrasted two traditions in medicine, personified in the classical myths of Hygiea and Asclepius:

> For the worshippers of Hygiea, health is the natural order of things, a positive attribute to which men are entitled if they govern their lives wisely. According to them, the most important function of medicine is to discover and teach the natural laws which will ensure to man a healthy mind in a healthy body.
>
> (Dubos 1960: 109)

On the other hand, stood the followers of Asclepius: 'more sceptical or wiser in the ways of the world', they believe that 'the chief role of the physician is to treat disease, to restore health by correcting any imperfection caused by the accidents of birth or of life.' Though Dubos has subsequently been celebrated as a critic of 'biomedicine' and as an advocate of the cult of Hygiea, this is a one-sided interpretation of his work. Indeed he explicitly repudiated the fantasy of 'harmonious equilibrium with nature' as 'an abstract concept with a Platonic beauty but lacking the flesh and blood of life' (Dubos 1960: 31). His argument was for recognition of the 'never ending oscillation between two different points of view in medicine' and of the need for a synthesis of both.

The key problem identified by Dubos was what became known in the 1970s as 'the epidemiological transition' (Omran 1971). Addel Omran, an American epidemiologist, offered a history of humanity in three ages: 'pestilence and famine' (life expectancy 20–40 years); 'receding pandemics' (life expectancy 30–50 years); 'degenerative and man-made diseases' (life expectancy more than 50 years). The 'pandemic' infectious diseases that had been the main cause of premature mortality, particularly among children and particularly in the cities created by modern industry, had declined in significance, largely as a result of improvements in sanitation and social conditions, partly as a result of immunisation and antibiotics. Contemporary Western society now faced quite different health problems: heart attacks, strokes and cancer were the major killers, especially of older people, and arthritis, diabetes, asthma were the major causes of ill health. In dealing with this new pattern of disease and disability, the methods of modern medicine appeared to be reaping diminishing returns.

One manifestation of the declining efficacy of modern medicine was a slowing in the pace of development of new drugs. According to one estimate, the rate of appearance of genuinely new drugs – rather than modifications of familiar products – declined from around 70 a year in the 1960s to less than 20 a year in the 1970s (Steward, Wibberley 1980). A related development was the recognition of an increasing range of side-effects of drugs that had recently come into use. The most disastrous of these was the sedative Thalidomide produced in Germany in 1956 and first prescribed in Britain two years later. By 1961 it was found to produce limb abnormalties in babies if taken during pregnancy, and it was withdrawn. There were also signs of a growing disillusionment with medical technology. The proliferation of high-tech 'coronary care units' in the 1970s was rapidly followed by research that showed that people had just as good a chance of survival if they stayed at home after a heart attack. In the USA, President Richard Nixon had declared 'war on cancer' in 1970, but survival rates remained substantially unchanged. Medical research in teaching hospitals was exposed and denounced as 'a vehicle for self-advancement rather than bettering the patient's condition' (Lock 1997: 136). In 1971, Macfarlane Burnet, Nobel laureate and founding father of immunology, offered a gloomy prognosis for the discipline he had done much to create, concluding that it had little potential for dealing with the new pattern of disease and arguing that the future lay in the social rather than the biological sciences (Burnet 1971).

Up to the early 1970s the problems of the epidemiological transition and the difficulties facing medical science remained for the most part matters of controversy within the world of medicine itself. However, these events unfolded in the context of major social changes affecting all Western societies. By the late 1960s the long post-war economic boom was coming to an end and in the early 1970s all Western economies went into recession, with the return of inflation and unemployment on a scale not seen since the 1930s. The resulting upsurge in trade union militancy in Europe was linked to a wider youthful radicalisation across the Western world, most conspicuously in the USA, where it was linked to causes of black civil rights, women's liberation and opposition to the Vietnam War.

From the late 1960s onwards, conditions of social stability and political consensus that had prevailed for more than two decades began to break down, with wide-ranging consequences, for doctors and health care systems as for other institutions in society. In terms of the effects of these social forces on medicine, the 1970s can be divided into two phases: an early radical, optimistic, phase and a later phase of conservative reaction in which a more pessimistic outlook became increasingly influential.

The radical challenge

One of the central principles of the radical upsurge symbolised by the May 1968 events in Paris was the commitment to self-expression and to the assertion of individuality against structures of society perceived as authoritarian and oppressive. In the USA, where the collectivist traditions still upheld by labour movements in Europe were conspicuously weak, and individualistic values were deeply rooted in popular culture, the youthful assertion of individuality took a particularly vigorous form. As the civil rights cause lost momentum as a protest movement in the 1970s, it offered a model for a range of 'new social movements' advocating the rights of women, students, gays, children, benefit claimants and many more. In what Starr characterised as a 'generalisation of rights' there was a dramatic expansion in both the 'variety and detail' of rights demanded:

> Medical care figured prominently in this generalisation of rights, particularly as a concern of the women's movement and in the new movements specifically for patients' rights and for the right of the handicapped, the mentally ill, the retarded and the subjects of medical experiments.
>
> (Starr 1982: 388)

The 'new social movements' demanded 'health care as a matter of right, not privilege: no other single idea so captures the spirit of the time' (Starr 1982: 389). No such right had ever been recognised in law, least of all in the USA, where access to health care was strictly controlled according either to the insurance principle or to strict eligibility criteria for state welfare services. Nevertheless, the claim for health care as a right was 'for a time so widely acknowledged as almost to be uncontroversial'. Given the universal access to health care offered by the NHS in Britain, the demand for health care as a right had little resonance. However, the wider demand for rights *in* health care, arising from a 'new self-assertiveness among the sick', soon became apparent on both sides of the Atlantic (Porter 1997: 689). This spirit was expressed in the emergence of self-help and pressure groups and in a general decline in deference to medical authority.

Two movements – feminism and 'anti-psychiatry' – were particularly influential in the growing challenge to the medical profession. Though these movements expressed an individualistic and consumerist perspective, both were associated with wider goals of personal and social liberation. These movements expressed the concerns of patients, but they also won some support among a younger generation of radical practitioners. They were also significant in linking the discontents of the world of medicine with those of the wider society.

The women's health movement criticised medical intervention in women's lives as paternalistic and patronising and particularly questioned doctors' control over pregnancy and childbirth, contraception and abortion. British feminist Ann Oakley provided a list of controversies over 'the modern male-controlled reproductive care system':

> These protests cover such topics as the undue use of surgical abortion techniques (as opposed to the safer and less traumatic suction method), the overuse of radical as opposed to conservative surgery for breast and reproductive tract diseases, the resistance of doctors to hormone replacement therapy for menopausal problems, inadequate attention paid to the psychological traumata of reproductive experiences, and, perhaps most central of all, the modern, male-controlled, hospitalized and increasingly technological pattern of child-birth management.
>
> (Oakley 1976: 52–3)

Oakley proceeded with a detailed indictment of virtually every aspect of the contemporary medical management of labour, from shaving and enemas to inductions, epidurals and Caesarians. She concluded by asserting that the political programme of the women's movement should include regaining control over reproductive care from doctors who had taken it out of the hands of midwives and other 'wise women'.

Self-help was an important principle of the new movement. The Boston Women's Health Collective handbook *Our Bodies Ourselves*, first circulated in a duplicated form in 1971 and published in 1972, rapidly made an international impact (Boston Women's Health Collective 1972). A *Women's Health Handbook*, subtitled 'a self-help guide', inspired by the Boston group, was published in Britain (MacKeith 1976). These guides included detailed advice on 'self-examination' (including the use of a vaginal speculum) and information about a wide range of women's health problems.

The anti-psychiatry movement drew support from a number of intellectual currents that emerged in the 1960s. Erving Goffman's *Asylums*, subtitled 'essays on the social situation of mental patients and other inmates', first published in 1961, was a powerful indictment of the dehumanising effect of the psychiatric hospital, based on his own anthropological fieldwork (Goffman 1961). Thomas Szasz, an American psychiatrist, with a right-wing libertarian outlook, wrote a number of provocatively titled books – such as *The Myth of Mental Illness* and the *The Manufacture of Madness* – in an increasingly outspoken challenge to the psychiatric mainstream (Szasz 1961, 1970). From a radical existentialist perspective the charismatic Scottish psychiatrist R.D. Laing argued in a number of works, starting from *The Divided Self* in 1960, that mental illness was more a socially-prescribed label than an objectively verifiable disease and that psychosis could be a process of healing that should not be suppressed by drugs (Laing 1960). In France, the philosopher Michel Foucault, best known for his historical studies of the role of psychiatric institutions in the social control processes of bourgeois society, also became associated with the anti-psychiatry movement (Foucault 1961).

In the course of the 1970s, the ideas of anti-psychiatry were taken up by movements both of and on behalf of people with a range of psychiatric problems. They also became an influential current in the wider radical counterculture (for a brilliant critique of these trends see Peter Sedgwick's *Psychopolitics*, 1982). Through television and film, they began to reach a much wider audience. In 1971 Ken Loach's *Family Life* presented Laing's theories on the causation of schizophrenia by dysfunctional family relationships. In 1975 Ken Kesey's novel *One Flew Over the Cuckoo's Nest*, which depicted psychiatric illness as a higher form of awareness and exposed the oppressive conditions of the mental hospital, was made into an award-winning film starring Jack Nicholson.

One common feature of the questioning of established medicine from different social movements was a challenge to the authority of the medical profession. The tendency for the demand for rights in the USA to lead to legal intervention in relations between patients and doctors had the effect of undermining professional sovereignty. Trust in medical authority was displaced by a conception of the doctor–patient relationship as a partnership in decision-making. Yet even in Britain, where litigation was a marginal influence, there was a shift in the perception from that of the doctor as an essentially benign figure, to one from whom the patient needed a degree of protection. Feminists were scathing: 'professionalism in medicine is nothing more than the institutionalisation of a male upper class monopoly' (Ehrenreich and English, 1974: 40). Left-wing commentators, particularly in America, exposed the 'medical-industrial complex', depicted the medical profession as an instrument of capitalist class rule and denounced 'medical ideology' (Navarro 1976; Waitzkin 1978). Commentators on medicine from other academic fields, formerly sympathetic towards doctors, increasingly 'portrayed the medical profession as a dominating, monopolising, self-interested force' (Starr, 1982: 392). Once a hero, the doctor had now become a villain.

The radical critics of medicine were often fiercely polemical, but like the wider movements of which they were a part, they were optimistic about their capacity to change things and not lacking in alternative programmes. Undoubtedly some of medicine's critics aspired to overthrow capitalism and patriarchy as well as the power of the medical profession, but many had more specific proposals for reform. Indeed some of these – such as demands for de-institutionalisation of treatment and care for the mentally ill and for the de-medicalisation of many aspects of childbirth – were rapidly assimilated by the mainstream. Pressures for reform of the American health-care system made some headway before becoming stalled in the complexities of the political process and its relations with doctors, insurers and other commercial interests. Parallel pressures for reform of the medical profession itself – notably in the recruitment of women – made steady progress. The proportion of women admitted to medical schools in Britain increased from 22 per cent in 1965–66, to 41 per cent in 1980–81 and reached 52 per cent in 1992–93 (Allen 1994).

The generalisation of doubt

In the late 1970s and early 1980s there was a marked change in the political mood of Western societies which had important consequences for the medical profession. In the recessionary climate of the mid-1970s the radical upsurge was gradually contained and a conservative backlash gathered momentum. By the end of the decade the new right was in the ascendant with Margaret Thatcher in 10 Downing Street and her ideological ally Ronald Reagan in the White House. The new conservatism did not however mean that doctors would be delivered from their carping critics and freed to return to business as usual. The end of the era of consensus led to a growing scepticism about the scope for ameliorative intervention in society, whether by the state or by professionals, whether in the spheres of education, social services or health. In a trend he dubbed 'the generalisation of doubt', Starr commented that the 'net effectiveness of the medical system as a whole was called into question' (Starr, 1982: 408). Far from being halted, the crisis of medical authority broadened and a more cynical attitude towards doctors became widespread.

The author who best exemplifies the nihilistic spirit of the late 1970s is Ivan Illich, a renegade Jesuit priest, who had already denounced the education system with his book *Deschooling Society*. In 1975 he published *Medical Nemesis*, the opening sentence of which declared that 'the medical establishment has become a major threat to health'. Illich incorporated the familiar criticisms (indeed, as we have seen above, self-criticisms) of modern medicine into his thesis that the health problems of society were predominantly those of 'iatrogenesis', illness caused by doctors. The result was 'the expropriation of man's coping ability by a maintenance service which keeps him geared up at the service of the industrial system' (Illich 1975: 160). The medical profession was a bureaucracy produced by an 'over-industrialised society'. Illich's vituperative polemic repudiated all piecemeal solutions: nothing less than the de-industrialisation of society and the de-bureaucratisation of medicine could save the world from medical nemesis: 'the inevitable punishment of inhuman attempts to be a hero rather than a human being' (Illich 1975: 28). For Illich, medical nemesis was 'resistant to medical care' and 'could be reversed only through a recovery of mutual self-care by the laity'.

The fact that such a bleak indictment of modern medicine could have a significant impact reflects the gloomy climate of the times. While few were prepared to go all the way with Illich's manifesto, it helped to encourage two trends which attracted growing support – the movement for a 'holistic' approach to health and the continuing offensive against the medical profession.

In his 1976 book *The role of medicine*, Thomas McKeown, professor of epidemiology at Birmingham, developed the arguments around the 'epidemiological transition', to which he had already made a substantial contribution, synthesised in *The modern rise of population* (McKeown 1976a, 1976b). To his earlier thesis that the contribution of medical science to the declining mortality from infectious disease was marginal compared with the role of improving social conditions and nutritional standards, McKeown now appended the view that the continuing focus of modern medicine on high-technology interventions aimed at curing disease was misplaced. He claimed that this approach had 'led to indifference to the external influences and personal behaviour which are the predominant determinants of health' (McKeown 1979: xvi). Though McKeown's thesis about the negligible medical contribution to the improved health of modern society was contested, it had a major impact: five years later a review of the literature accurately noted that 'McKeown's views have been so immensely influential that they have almost become a new orthodoxy' (Davey *et al.* 1984: 179).

McKeown's contention that modern medicine treated the human body 'as a machine' struck a chord at a time when an anti-technological and environmentalist outlook was becoming increasingly popular. Though McKeown was careful to distinguish between the role of medicine as an institution, which he questioned, and clinical practice, of which he broadly approved, his balanced approach was not shared by many of his readers who interpreted his work as a categorical repudiation of scientific medicine. It was striking that in the second edition of *The Role of Medicine*, he felt obliged to include a preface distancing himself from Illich and from those who had interpreted his book as 'an attack on clinical medicine' (McKeown 1979: vii). Notwithstanding McKeown's misgivings, there can be little doubt that the popularity of his work reflected the growing influence of an ecological consciousness that upheld a 'holistic' alternative to the 'biomedical' tradition. The growing popularity of diverse forms of 'alternative' and 'complementary' medicine confirmed the growing disillusionment with orthodox medicine.

Another theme of Illich's that also appeared in McKeown's work was that of the role of 'personal behaviour' in the genesis of modern health problems. At a time when governments were preoccupied with curbing public expenditure and ideologues of the new right were promoting notions of individual responsiblity, it was not surprising that there was considerable enthusiasm for the legitimation of these notions in terms of health. In 1977 the American neoconservative political scientist Aaron Wildavsky presented an appraisal of the crisis of medicine to a symposium sponsored by the Rockefeller Foundation, a right-wing think tank, under the title 'Doing Better and Feeling Worse' (Wildavsky, 1977). Another contribution, from John Knowles, president of the foundation, called for a greater emphasis on changing individual behaviour (Knowles 1977). In the long-running argument between radicals, who emphasised the contribution of social factors to health, and conservatives, who focused on individual responsibility, the wider balance of forces in society shifted the consensus inexorably towards the right.

The anti-professional bandwagon also gathered momentum. While earlier criticisms had come from radicals and feminists, the ranks of the enemies of the medical profession now widened to include mainstream academics and media commentators. In 1980 academic lawyer and moral philosopher Ian Kennedy devoted his Reith Lectures to a systematic onslaught on doctors, subsequently published as *The unmasking of medicine* (1981). His central argument was that the ascendancy of a mechanistic conception of the body had resulted in modern medicine becoming positively damaging to the health and well-being of the population. Whereas McKeown had tried to distance himself from Illich, Kennedy credited both among his principal sources and recycled their main arguments.

Two key themes emerged from Kennedy's diatribe. One was 'the need for each person to take greater responsibility for his own life, which includes his health' (Kennedy 1981: ix). As we have seen, this became a familiar feature of government policy in the 1980s and 1990s. The second was the promotion of a 'consumerist' challenge to the professional self-regulation of doctors, whom he accused of 'stubborn intransigence' in face of proposals for reform. Now, declared Kennedy, 'consumerism must take another tack': 'A wholly new system of supervision and sanction must be created, with the power to suspend the incompetent or even remove from practice those found to merit it.' (Kennedy 1981: 139). It took another 20 years before Kennedy's proposals in this area began to be implemented; in 1998 he was appointed chairman of the independent inquiry into the scandal at the children's heart surgery unit in Bristol.

It was not surprising that, by the late 1970s, the medical profession was beginning to show signs of strain. Colin Dollery, professor of clinical pharmacology at the Royal Postgraduate Medical School, looked back wistfully on the golden age of post-war drug research and development (in which he had played a leading role) and concluded that we had reached *The end of an age of optimism* (Dollery 1978). Even some of medicine's critics became concerned about what appeared to be an excessively gloomy outlook: 'from the belief that medicine can do everything, opinion is in danger of swinging to the equally untenable conclusion that it can do little or nothing' (McKeown, 1979: 178). Starr noted the paradox that an extreme cynicism about medicine and the medical profession had become widespread 'at a time when America is making exceptional advances in health' (Starr 1982: 410). The birth of the world's first test-tube baby in 1978 confirmed that (fairly basic) technology could still yield dramatic results. The discovery, by Australian gastroenterologist Barry Marshall, of the role of Helicobacter pylori infection in peptic ulcer showed that there was life left in the old germ theory. But even these advances could not stem the tide of public opprobrium. 'Just as medicine used to be uncritically given credit for gains in health that had other causes, so medicine was now disparaged without prudent regard for its benefits' (Starr 1982: 410).

Yet the medical profession survived the 1980s. It had sustained a significant loss of prestige and a decline in morale, but it still retained substantial authority in society. Bolstered, despite all its critics, by continuing advances in medical science and technology, medicine remained high in public regard and doctors were still widely respected. Though the medical profession may not have been as highly esteemed as in the past, other professions – in law, education, the church, not to mention politicians and journalists – had fared even worse. It was also noteworthy that, despite the growing number and influence of its detractors, the medical profession emerged remarkably unscathed from its political conflicts in the 1980s. In the USA, doctors succeeded in fighting off attempts by the insurance companies, health corporations and the government to reform the financing of health care. In Britain, the popularity of the NHS provided some defence for the medical profession against Mrs Thatcher's reforming zeal and doctors succcessfully subverted the first wave of managerial reform foisted on the NHS in the shape of the former Sainsbury's boss, Roy Griffiths (Hunter 1994).

The medical profession emerged from the 1980s battered, but with the basic structure and institutions built up over the previous 150 years intact. However, the events of the next decade would reveal the extent of internal decay concealed by the appearances of continuity.

Medicine's velvet revolution

The last decade of the twentieth century was a period of dramatic change in society and perhaps even more dramatic changes in the medical profession. By the turn of the millennium deeply-rooted traditions, such as those of self-regulation and the independent contractor status of GPs, had effectively been abandoned. Fundamental changes had been introduced in medical education and training, linked to changes in the place of medical science in medical practice and in the nature of the doctor/patient relationship. What was perhaps most remarkable was that there was little resistance to these revolutionary changes and indeed little comment upon them at all.

The breaching of the Berlin Wall on New Year's Eve 1989 was a highly symbolic event. It followed the collapse, one by one, of the Soviet-sponsored regimes of Eastern Europe, and it anticipated the collapse of the Soviet Union itself, in 1992. It marked the end of the world order established after the Second World War and consolidated through forty years of Cold War. Long fundamental divisons – between East and West in foreign affairs, between Left and Right at home – rapidly lost their force. The collapse of ancient polarities was linked to the decline of familiar collectivities (classes, unions, political parties, churches) and to the exhaustion of ideologies (socialism, communism, nationalism, even conservatism). In 1989 capitalism and liberal democracy claimed victory, but their triumphalism was always muted and the celebrations proved short-lived as the 1990s came to be dominated by preoccupations about the social and environmental dangers of globalised economic forces.

In an era of lowered horizons and diminished expectations a climate of scepticism about established forms of expertise – in science and technology, in politics and academic life, in traditional professions and institutions – became widespread. People became sceptical, not only about particular sources of authority, but in general, about the possibility of expertise in any area, especially in relation to any social or political objective. This was not a radical outlook, that was critical of the way things were from a perspective of how they might be changed for the better. It was a fatalistic one, which was cynical about the way things were because it had drawn the gloomy conclusion from the experience of the twentieth century that any attempt to change things could only make them worse.

The changes that were implemented in medicine in the course of the 1990s originated in a section of the medical elite. The old structures were overthrown by a movement initiated from above, not by a revolt from below. In this respect there is also a striking parallel with the 'velvet revolutions' of Eastern Europe: like the Stalinist bureaucracies, the old medical elite experienced an internal moral collapse and was replaced by a new clique emerging largely from its own ranks, drawing in some new blood and winning widespread approval from the younger generation in the profession. A series of events in the early 1990s signalled the capitulation of the old order and the ascendancy of the new. One was the shift in the medical attitude towards non-orthodox therapies as the traditional concern to uphold scientific principles and maintain a clear demarcation was displaced by a more open and collaborative approach. This shift was symbolised by the reversal in the BMA line in its 1993 report on 'complementary medicine'. Another key change was heralded by the publication of the GMC's *Tomorrow's Doctors* in 1993: after decades of stasis a major reform of medical education was not only announced, but rapidly implemented. The quest for reassurance about the quality of medical practice was expressed in the pursuit of various forms of audit and in the adoption of guidelines in different areas of clinical practice. These methods became widespread in the early 1990s and towards the end of the decade were absorbed into the framework of managerial control known as 'clinical govern-ance'. Let's look at each of these areas more closely.

From 'alternative therapy' to 'complementary medicine'

The contrast between the BMA's 1993 report and one produced only seven years earlier on the same subject, entitled *Alternative Therapy*, is dramatic. 'During the Prince of Wales' term as President of the BMA (1982–83)', notes the introduction to the earlier report, 'he urged the Association to look critically at modern medicine' (BMA 1986: 1). In response the BMA established a working party, which produced its report in 1986. The report expressed a distinctly curmudgeonly attitude to what its authors clearly regarded as the Prince's rather tiresome hobbyhorse. It recognised an 'identifiable growth of an underlying hostility to technology and science, allied to a distrust of innovation' from which 'orthodox medicine' was not immune (BMA 1986: 3). With some disdain, the BMA noted 'a demand which is scarcely rational for instant cures for the currently incurable diseases of mankind' and dismissed the 'ill-founded suspicion that nothing is being done to attack these problems' (BMA 1986: 4). In a tone of increasing rancour, the report warned of the danger of 'turning back to primitive beliefs and outmoded practices, almost all purposeless and without a sound base, however well-meaning'.

The BMA first offered a lengthy history and defence of the traditions of scientific medicine, taking up about one third of the report. Only then did it provide a series of (overwhelmingly disparaging) assessments of a range of alternative therapies, including acupuncture and homeopathy, herbalism and hypnotherapy. It concluded that these and many other therapies had 'little in common between them, except that they pay little regard to the scientific principles of orthodox medicine' (BMA 1986: 77). The report emphasised that the 'fundamental division' separating orthodox and alternative approaches was 'the scientific principle which underlies the former, and the testing of theories by systematic observation which that principle implies':

> The steadily developing body of orthodox medical knowledge, based on science, has led to large, demonstrable, and reproducible benefits for mankind, on a scale which the alternative approach cannot match.
>
> (BMA 1986: 78)

The BMA report acknowledged that part of the appeal of alternative practitioners was the time and compassion they were able to offer to their patients, but insisted that this was also an important feature of good orthodox practice, which was 'sometimes limited by the pressures of work'. It also acknowledged that medical development had in the past been assisted by concepts and techniques derived from unorthodox sources, but emphasised that these must be evaluated by 'systematic, scientific' methods before they could be incorporated into the mainstream.

By the evidence of this report, in the mid-1980s mainstream medicine was confident about the methods and proud of the achievements of medical science and unwilling to make any concessions to unorthodox alternatives, even at the behest of the royal patron of the BMA. Before long it was singing a different tune.

In 1993, the BMA published *Complementary Medicine: New Approaches to Good Practice*, the product of another working party set up in response to the growing popularity of alternative therapies and to indications that medical attitudes to them were softening. A major survey of doctors undertaken by the BMA in 1992 revealed that 29 per cent of respondents believed that acupuncture and osteopathy should be provided in GPs' surgeries (37 per cent were opposed). Women GPs and those under 45 were more likely to be in favour of alternative approaches. The new report, which made only one passing reference to the 1986 report, adopted a much more conciliatory tone. In place of the previous spirited argument for scientific medicine, the new report offered a pragmatic, defensive, definition of 'conventional medicine' as 'that treatment which is delivered by a registered medical practitioner' (BMA 1993: 7). In a new posture of abject relativism, the BMA now proposed the term 'non-conventional therapies' as 'a general and neutral term within which to explore the diverse nature of different practices' (BMA 1993: 8).

Whereas a few years earlier the BMA had been concerned to draw a line of principle between orthodox and alternative therapies, it now sought to make a pragmatic distinction between different forms of non-conventional treatment. Having abandoned a definition of mainstream medical practice in terms of medical science, the BMA now decided that five complementary therapies – acupuncture, chiropractic, herbalism, homeopathy and osteopathy – could be regarded as 'discrete clinical disciplines'. This arbitrary classification was clearly based on judgements about which therapies were more popular (with patients and doctors) and were more established in terms of training and procedures of professional regulation. There was no attempt to make any objective claim for the superiority of, say homeopathy and herbalism over rolfing and iridiology. The BMA's main concern was to foster the professionalisation of the big five complementary therapies and to marginalise the rest. The price paid by the medical profession for this opportunist approach towards alternative therapies was to betray the historic commitment to medical science which had been the foundation of its growing success over two centuries.

It is quite understandable that patients who find conventional medicine ineffective and conventional medical practitioners unsympathetic should turn to alternative practitioners. But for orthodox doctors to collaborate with such practitioners implies a capitulation to irrationalism. Nor can the legitimacy of alternative therapeutic systems be enhanced by studies in the form of clinical trials which claim to show their effectiveness. No doubt many patients derive much therapeutic benefit from praying to statues and icons, but this is no reason why these techniques should be incorporated into clinical practice. In his commentary on the nineteenth century triumph of medical science over the antecedents of today's alternative therapies, Dalrymple observed that the distinctive feature of scientific medicine was its openness to critical evaluation, revision and improvement, features it shared with the wider Enlightenment traditions of reason and progress from which it emerged (Dalrymple 1998: 58). By contrast, rival approaches – such as Samuel Hahnemann's 'intellectually ridiculous' homeopathy – offered no comparable method of development, but were presented as 'complete, fully-formed' systems. The correspondence between the inquisitive and interventionist outlook of medical science and the dynamic and progressive values of Victorian Britain was the key to the early success of the medical profession.

Dumbing down

In *Tomorrow's Doctors*, the GMC outlined the 'goals and objectives' of the new curriculum under the rubric of 'knowledge, skills and attitudes' (GMC 1993). Whereas in the past knowledge was crammed for exams, skills were picked up on the job, and attitudes (for better or for worse) unconsciously assimilated, now students were going to be taught formally in all three areas. Knowledge would be reduced to a 'factual quantum' defined by a 'core curriculum': this would include the familiar basic medical sciences, but also unfamiliar subjects such as 'human relationships' and 'the importance of communication'. The extensive and detailed attitudinal objectives reflected the values of the culture of therapy and the demands of political correctness (neither previously a major influence on the medical mainstream). Students would be expected to show respect for patients' diverse identities and rights, they should be able to 'cope with uncertainty' and they should display an 'awareness of personal limitations, a willingness to seek help when necessary and an ability to work effectively as a member of a team'.

One of the key concepts of the new curriculum is that of 'problem-based' learning: instead of acquiring a grounding in basic medical sciences before encountering sick patients, students begin from a clinical problem presented by a patient and organise their studies around this problem (Lowry 1993: 28–32). The idea is that, by being relevant to the resolution of a real clinical problem, their study of anatomy, physiology, biochemistry, etc. will be more interesting and better retained. The role of the teacher is no longer to transmit knowledge, but to facilitate the process of problem-solving by students, working collectively, in teams.

The defect of problem-based learning is that it assumes that defining a clinical problem is a straightforward matter, whereas in practice it is often profoundly difficult. According to Abraham Flexner, whose historic 1910 report promoted the reorganisation of medical education in the USA on the basis of scientific medicine, 'for the analysis of the simplest situation which the ailing body presents, considerable knowledge is required' (Flexner 1925: 13) Furthermore, for practical treatment 'still another volume of knowledge and experience is requisite'. Flexner explicitly rejected the method of proceeding on 'superficial or empirical lines' which is what is implied by the notion of the 'relevance' of scientific inquiries to the problem that has been identified. It is a commonplace that what appears to be relevant or important to the untrained eye is revealed by science to be merely a manifestation of some underlying phenomenon. Indeed, if what appears to be relevant coincided with what is actually important, then there would be no need for science.

Flexner offered a definition of science as the 'persistent effort of men to purify, extend and organise their knowledge of the world in which they live' (Flexner 1925: 3). He particularly emphasised the word 'effort', insisting that students should 'strive to transcend native powers, prejudices, limitations'. This approach stands in sharp contrast to that of the new curriculum, in which the preoccupation with 'relevance' means elevating 'native powers, prejudices and limitations' over the systematic process of 'observation, inference, verification and generalisation' regarded by Flexner as the essence of the scientific method. For today's medical teachers, students should find the course 'enjoyable' and be allowed to study at 'their own pace and in their own time' rather than being expected to make an effort to transcend their own limitations (Dent, 1993). More than a decade earlier in the USA, Lewis Thomas had warned against 'notions of relevance' that were 'paralysing the minds of today's first year medical students' (Thomas 1979: 141).

The very fact that the medical curriculum has been repeatedly criticised for more than a century on the grounds that it is overloaded with facts – a period in which the 'facts' have changed considerably – suggests that this is a misconceived criticism. It implies a conception of medical science as a vast corpus of knowledge which has steadily increased in volume; from this perspective, medical education is a process of cramming all these facts into the student cranium. This approach confuses the process of scientific inquiry with its results: medical science is a method of understanding human health and disease, not a body of facts. The Nobel laureate Peter Medawar dismissed problems arising from the apparently 'oceanic volume of scientific knowledge' as 'essentially technological problems, for which adequate technological solutions are rapidly being found' (Medawar 1986: 70). And this was before electronic data bases, CD-ROMs and the internet. As Flexner wrote, 'the teacher cannot provide the student with bits of information likely to be useful, nor can study be prolonged to include everything' (Flexner 1925: 13). The increase in the scale of medical knowledge over the past century makes no qualitative difference to this judgement. The key issue was not facts, but 'habituation to method'; the role of the teacher was to select knowledge to exemplify scientific procedure. He insisted that 'the facts in question cannot be passively learned and mechanically applied' (Flexner 1925: 13). The object of medical education was 'primarily the effort to train students in the intellectual technique of inductive science' This required 'an extraordinarily active and oft-repeated mental process, involving observation, sorting out, combining, inferring, trying'.

The real problem of medical teaching over the years has not been a surfeit of facts but a deficit of training in the intellectual technique of inductive science. Unfortunately, the promoters of the new curriculum have responded to popular criticisms of 'overload' by replacing inductive science with a vulgar empiricism. Medical science is disparaged as 'knowledge' and reduced to easily assimilated fragments of a 'core' curriculum, according to the criteria of relevance and enjoyability. The main concern of medical schools has shifted towards the inculcation of what are considered to be the correct attitudes. The Oxford physician David Weatherall is one of the few leading medical figures to have pointed – in a strikingly tentative way – to the dangers of this approach:

> While the motives behind these changes are admirable, it is essential that, while trying to improve the social, pastoral and communication skills of our future doctors, we do not dilute their scientific education.
>
> (Weatherall, 1995: 329)

One of the most significant innovations of the new curriculum is the introduction of formal teaching for medical students in communication skills. Indeed such teaching has extended rapidly into the post-graduate domain and into the 'continuing medical education' of practising doctors. Inadequacies in communication skills are one of the most frequently cited problems of 'poorly performing doctors' and the provision of appropriate tuition in this area is one of the functions of the 'assessment and support centres' proposed by the government.

To anybody who has encountered a doctor who was rude or patronising or who spoke in incomprehensible medical jargon (and anecdotal evidence suggests that these are all familiar experiences) it would seem a good idea that medical students should be taught how to communicate with their future patients. But is it possible to teach communication skills? In one widely used set of guidelines on communication, there is a striking combination of the most elementary 'basic steps' and suggestions about profoundly difficult matters such as 'responding to patient feelings' (Buckman 1994). No doubt it is possible to instruct students in 'basic steps', such as the importance of introductions, shaking hands, sitting down, listening attentively, etc. Perhaps in the past such conduct would have been regarded as simple good manners, which students might have been expected to acquire at home rather than at medical school. However, it may be fairly argued that the manifest lack of such elementary civility towards their patients among many doctors justifies including such instruction in the curriculum. Nevertheless, it is difficult to imagine that it would be necessary to spend more than a few minutes in an overcrowded curriculum on such tuition.

When it comes to communications between doctors and patients at a higher level of subtlety, which rely on establishing a degree of empathy, and are heavily influenced by the past record of mutual experience and trust, it is doubtful whether formal instruction, whether in the form of books, videos or role-playing can be of much assistance. Such skills fall into the category of things that can be learned by observation and reflection in clinical situations, not taught in a classroom (McCormick 1996). Indeed the very attempt to teach them in such a formal way underestimates the subtleties of doctor–patient communication which generations of doctors have painstakingly acquired through the sort of apprenticeship experience that is now so disparaged. The net effect of the promotion of comic-book communication skills is to elevate the banal while degrading what is profound in medical practice (Willis 1995: 127).

Clinical governance

Clinical governance means the extension into the medical world of new mechanisms of regulation through audit that have been developed in business. These amount, according to Michael Power, professor of accountancy at the London School of Economics, to 'the spread of a distinct mentality of administrative control, a pervasive logic which has a life of its own over and above specific practices' (Power 1994). Power describes an 'audit explosion' in the late 1980s and early 1990s, as the term 'began to be used in Britain with growing frequency in a wide variety of contexts' (Power 1997: 3). A perception of a general deterioration in professional confidence and public trust in business and in services, in both private and public sectors, resulted in a quest for external guarantees of quality and probity. But audit is not a neutral process: when people subject their work to external monitoring, they inevitably find that this process leads to a reorganisation of their work to comply with the requirements of audit. As Power writes, 'audit is not simply a solution to a technical problem; it also makes possible ways of redesigning the process of government' (Power 1997: 11).

Though audit is designed to reassure, Power argues that it has ambivalent implications for relations of trust. Where trust is lacking, people hope that it can be restored through audit. But can you trust the auditor? The audit society tends to create 'an inflationary spiral' of trust in more remote sources of reassurance, or to put it another way, it fosters increasing distrust:

> Assumptions of distrust sustaining audit processes may be self-fulfilling as auditees adapt their behaviour strategically in response to the audit process, thereby becoming less trustworthy.
>
> (Power 1997: 136)

The net result may be that the quality of service is damaged even though the goals of efficiency, or cost-effectiveness are achieved.

In a detailed study of the impact of the ideology of audit on the world of health, Power notes that this has created 'an enormous environmental disturbance' (Power 1997: 108). He comments on the attempt to adapt medical audit to managerial purposes that this 'fragile practice' was 'never intended as a public accountability device' (Power 1997:109). As medical audit has been assimilated into clinical governance, concerns about the quality of patient care have become subordinate to the managerial performance imperatives. Power concludes that faith in audit as a means of regulating medical performance reflects wider social anxieties, affecting doctors and patients as well as managers and politicians, and the 'need to create images of control in the face of risk' (Power 1997: 121). Other commentators have warned that this process may have adverse effects producing 'inspection overload' and irrevocable damage to cultures of trust (Day, Klein 1990).

The processes of clinical governance are not only time-consuming, but potentially demoralising, as the presence of a shadowy third party in doctor–patient relations has a subtly corrosive effect on professional authority. (Indeed this presence may not be so shadowy if proposals to video consultations as part of the revalidation process gain acceptance.) A number of commentators have drawn attention to the negative effects of the culture of guidelines on medical morale (Goodman 1998). Some have expressed concerns that guidelines can stifle innovation and encourage defensive practice (this is certainly likely to increase if departures from national guidelines become the basis for litigation) (Fletcher, Fletcher 1990). Others fear that 'insufficient attention will be paid to the sometimes nebulous concepts of trust and culture in a headlong rush for the more tangible appeals of measurement, monitoring and coercive control mechanisms' (Davies, Mannion 1999).

In a brief commentary on 'the perils of checklist medicine', London GP Iona Heath has pointed out some of the dangers of the preoccupation with guidelines on doctor–patient relationships (Heath 1995). As she observes, 'guidelines are constructed from evidence from research derived from studies of populations and are predicated on the notion of a composite patient which may have little immediate relevance to the troubled person who presents in the consulting room'. She warns that guidelines 'depersonalise individual patients and turn them into diseases' and that the managerial use of guidelines to monitor practice 'implies levels of coercion and control which are potentially destructive of the fragile good that is the doctor–patient relationship'.

Revalidation

The proposed system of revalidation will have far-reaching consequences for the professional standing of doctors and for our relations with our patients. For GPs, it will take the form of 'a continuous process with an episodic submission and assessment of fitness to continue in general practice' (RCGP November 1999: 5). Assessment will take place against detailed standards of acceptable and unacceptable conduct under the headings of 'professional competence', 'good relations with patients and colleagues' and 'professional ethical obligations' (RCGP October 1999: 1). But why is such a drastic change necessary, and why now? The immediate response to these questions from supporters of the new system is that the proposed reforms are necessary to restore public confidence in doctors and the NHS in response to 'a progression of "rogue dotors" and health care scandals through the media' (Smith 1999). But the problem of 'under-performing' doctors is not new: there have always been idle and incompetent doctors, just as there have always been some who who have succumbed to the temptations of alcohol and drugs, lust and lucre and other forms of corruption. I have seen no convincing evidence that the scale of these problems has increased in recent years – and my strong personal impression is that, at least among GPs, both the intensity of work and the level of medical competence have increased substantially.

Advocates of the new system point to a wider breakdown of trust in relations between doctors and patients and to a loss of public confidence in the medical profession and in its mechanisms of self-regulation. In fact, surveys reveal remarkably high levels of popular respect for the medical profession: a MORI poll in January 1999 revealed that 91 per cent of the public trusted doctors to tell the truth (an increase from 86 per cent in 1997 and 82 per cent in 1983) whereas only 80 per cent trusted vicars (BMA January 1999). A follow up poll in March 2000, after the Shipman verdict, revealed that 87 per cent still trusted doctors to tell the truth (confidence in vicars had fallen to 78 per cent, slightly higher than judges at 77 per cent) (*BMJ* 2000, 320: 653). Furthermore an official government survey of general practice patients in 1998 revealed a high level of satisfaction with the service, most notably in the sphere of doctor–patient communication: 94 per cent of respondents said that their GP was very or fairly easy to under-stand; 87 per cent said that all, or almost all, of the time they were given enough information about their treatment (DoH 1998b). The greatly exaggerated perception (among doctors) of their loss of prestige reflects the underlying force driving this process forward: the crisis of confidence of the medical profession itself.

In invoking public demand for tighter regulation, the leaders of the medical profession have projected their own insecurities into society. To the extent that there is popular support for measures such as revalidation, it has largely been fostered by leading medical figures, such as GMC president Donald Irvine, in their responses to scandals such as Bristol and the Shipman case. The danger of the revalidation proposals is that they will exacerbate the medical profession's loss of confidence rather than alleviating it. The problem is not merely that the drive towards revalidation will lead to the creation of scapegoats and a spate of early retirements, though it undoubtedly will. There is an even more serious danger that it will degrade the profession as a whole and do further damage to the relationship between doctor and patient.

9

CONCLUSION

In May 1999, the BMA called for a moratorium on the commercial farming of genetically-modified (GM) crops until there was a 'scientific consensus' on their safety. This statement followed a series of incidents in which environmental protestors had destroyed experimental GM projects and a media campaign for a ban on further developments. The BMA demanded that 'the precautionary principle should be applied in developing modified crops or foodstuffs, as we cannot at present know whether there are any serious risks to the environment or to human health involved in producing GM crops or consuming GM food products'. (BMA 1999: 12). The government, squeezed between a recognition of the substantial economic potential of GM products and mounting public anxieties, tried to hold the line. In May the government's Chief Scientist (Robert May) and Chief Medical Officer (Liam Donaldson) issued a joint statement reassuring the public that there was 'no current evidence to suggest that the process of genetic modification is inherently harmful'. In early 2000, however, the government crumbled and announced even tighter restrictions on the development of GM foodstuffs.

In his classic text, *The Mirage of Health*, published forty years before the GM controversy, Rene Dubos noted the widespread conviction that maintaining the scientific status quo would safeguard humanity against new threats: 'It is often suggested that a moratorium on science would give mankind the opportunity to search its soul and discover a solution to the problems that threaten its very survival' (Dubos 1960: 214). He commented that 'this static formula of survival' was 'not new': 'indeed it has been used with much biological success by social insects'. Through a highly stratified and efficient mode of organisation, colonies of ants and termites had solved many of the problems which were the subject of

155

endless discussions and conflicts in human societies. In a similar way, the 'arrested societies' of isolated aboriginal groups, which 'resembled in some respects the societies of bees and ants', confirmed the possibility of achieving a stable equilibrium with their environment – and 'an acceptable degree of physical health and happiness'. However, though this stability may have allowed these societies to avoid the problems of adapting to change, it was also 'incompatible with the growth of their civilisations, indeed, with the very growth of man' (Dubos 1960: 215).

The approval of a moratorium on the development of GM food because of possible dangers to health, by prestigious bodies of the medical profession and the scientfic community as well as by the government, is a reflection of the fatalistic outlook of contemporary society. In the current climate, every scientific advance, from test-tube babies to key-hole surgery, provokes more anxiety at the possible adverse consequences than celebration of the potential benefits. Fears about the dangers of science are part of a wider pessimism about the prospects for the advance of humanity through active intervention in nature or in society (Gillott, Kumar 1995). Though the rising influence of environmentalism has not yet led to the promotion of insect colonies as a model for human society, the popular cult of the primitive (as reflected, for example, in the affinity of contemporary environmentalists for the tribal peoples of the rainforests) indicates the scale of disillusionment with achievements of civilisation (Bookchin 1995). Given the impracticability of a return to an idealised aboriginal state, this outlook is expressed in demands to call a halt to further attempts at human advance, whether through scientific or social initiatives. In a society of lowered horizons and diminished expectations, security and safety have become the highest values and the goal of preserving health has become the zenith of human aspirations.

The idea that to safeguard health it is necessary to restrain, if not stop, scientific advance appears to be in stark contrast to the widely quoted utopian concept of health adopted by the World Health Organisation at its founding conference in 1946: 'Health is a state of complete physical, mental and social well-being, and not merely the absence of disease or infirmity' (MacKenzie 1946) Yet, as Dubos observed, dreams of an imaginary past and utopian visions of the future share a common theme: 'different as they appear to be, both imply a static view of the world which is incompatible with reality, for the human condition has always been to move on' (Dubos 1960: 208). It is striking that, after its adoption in that brief period of hope for the future between the end of the Second World War in 1945 and the onset of the Cold War in 1947, the WHO's definition of health disappeared from public view until it was rediscovered in the 1970s. If, as Dubos noted, myths of a golden age provide mankind with 'solace in times of despair and with elan during the expansive periods of history', then we can readily identify the heady days of post-war reconstruction with the latter, and the period of increasing gloom that began with the recession of the 1970s with the former.

The defect of utopian visions and static formulas is that they are out of tune with that restless quest for change which distinguishes humanity from the rest of the natural world:

> Life is an adventure in a world where nothing is static; where unpredictable and ill-understood events constitute dangers that must be overcome, often blindly and at great cost; where man, like the sorceror's apprentice, has set in motion forces that are potentially dangerous and may some day escape his control.
>
> (Dubos 1960: 11)

For Dubos, disease was an inescapable manifestation of the life of adventure and struggle through which humanity extended its creative potential. Far from being an end in itself, health was 'the condition best suited to reach goals that each individual formulates for himself', in a process guided by social rather than biological urges (Dubos 1960: 219). Writing in more optimistic times, he recognised that the pursuit of certain human ideals and goals may have unfavourable consequences for the human species, but accepted that this was a price that must be paid for progress. As he emphasised, 'it is man's dignity to value certain ideals above comfort, and even above life'. Indeed it is this human trait that makes medicine a philosophy that goes beyond the conception of man as a living machine to encompass 'the collective aspirations of mankind'. From this perspective, a 'perfect policy of public health' is possible for a colony of insects or a herd of cows, but not for man: 'human life implies adventure, and there is no adventure without struggles and dangers'.

CONCLUSION

Health and the end of history

The rise of health to become one of the central goals of human endeavour over the past decade reflects the peculiar stasis of modern society. In the widely acclaimed formulation of one contemporary historian, the parallel triumphs of the West over the East, the free market over the planned economy, marked 'the end of history' (Fukuyama 1989). Yet, far from inaugurating a new era of social harmony, the victory of capitalism rapidly revealed the profound exhaustion of its ideologues and a sense that their system too had reached the end of the road (Furedi 1992). It appeared that this victory, the outcome of more than a century of more or less intense class conflicts fought on both international and domestic fronts, had been bought at a high cost. In discrediting the goals of communism, any concept of social progress had been put in question. In challenging the values of socialism, the bourgeois principles of liberty and equality had also been disowned. In rolling back the menace of the Russian Revolution, the achievements of the French Revolution too were repudiated. In disputing the possibility of the constructive human intervention in nature and society, the scientific principles of the Enlightenment, indeed the claims of rationality itself, came under deep suspicion. The weary, nihilistic outlook of post-modernism that became increasingly influential in pre-millennial Western society reflected a loss of conviction in history as a human-centred project.

Despite claims that history had come to an end, society has not in fact stood still – indeed many have experienced change in a more intense way than ever before. But change in the modern world no longer appears to be the outcome of conscious human direction or purpose – it appears as the unpredictable outcome of the random, chaotic actions of diverse, isolated individuals and uncontrollable social (and natural) forces. Not surprisingly, change perceived in this way provokes fear and anxiety rather than any positive sense of anticipation about the future, let alone any inclination to play an active role in influencing its character. The perception of society as both out of control and increasingly unstable leads to a heightened consciousness of the risks of everyday life and an intensified awareness of ubiquitous threats to health (Beck 1992). The fear of risks and dangers results in both self-imposed restrictions on personal behaviour and in an acceptance of externally-dictated limits on the scope of human activity. Anthony Giddens, sociologist and intellectual guide to New Labour, celebrated the emergence of risk as a force of moral regulation: 'We can't return to nature or to tradition, but, individually and as collective humanity, we can seek to remoralise our lives in the context of a positive acceptance of manufactured uncertainty' (Giddens 1994: 227). A sense of low expectations has converged with a heightened sense of risk to restrict the scope of individual activity and diminish our common humanity.

The impasse reached by Western society in the 1990s was experienced differently by different sections of society. Perceptions were strongly influenced by parallel economic and social developments, in particular by the demise of traditional forms of collectivity and the accelerated erosion of familiar institutions, from the Royal Family to the nuclear family. The decline of old-style class conflict brought an end to long-established patterns of industrial and political conflict. It also removed a key source of cohesion on both sides of the great divide, compounding wider atomising forces to produce an unprecedented degree of individuation in society. If the proletarian solidarity of the trade unions and the labour movement effectively disintegrated, so too did the spirit of class loyalty that had made the Conservative Party such a successful social movement.

'The toffs have opted out' noted Alan Clark, once a minister under Mrs Thatcher, in his notorious diaries (Clark 1994). For this cynical aristocrat, the loss of nerve of the upper crust clique, which had always informally appointed the leader of the Conservative Party, was revealed in the debacle which resulted in the replacement of Mrs Thatcher by John Major in November 1990. The abdication of leadership by the traditional elite of British society has become increasingly apparent throughout society, from industry and commerce to culture and services. In the business enterprise, it became standard practice for directors to defer to management consultants, public relations experts and ethical investment advisers. In a similar spirit of uncertainty, employers called in facilitators and counsellors to deal with workplace conflicts, drew up mission statements in an attempt to discover a sense of purpose, used codes of conduct to regulate working relationships and charters to appeal to customers. In the professions, the crisis of confidence was expressed in the quest for new forms of reassurance through audit, inspection and reaccreditation. In medicine, as we have seen, this has led to the emergence of guidelines, evidence-based medicine, clinical governance and revalidation. It has also encouraged a major expansion of the sphere of medical ethics, as doctors refer decisions in what were formerly regarded as clinical matters to ethical committees (and even to the courts).

One paradox of modern society is that, though intellectuals may dispute the possibility of scientific objectivity, entrepreneurs cannot run their production lines, or distribute and sell their goods and services, without the benefit of technology. Thus, technologicial development continues despite the stagnation of intellectual life. However, though there are still many people who are committed to experimentation and innovation, the prevailing climate is suspicious if not hostile to such activities, inducing a remarkably diffident outlook. Scientists, particularly those working in politically sensitive areas such as genetics, are reluctant to take responsibility for their own work, preferring to invite some external agency to regulate it.

For the mass of people, the main effect of the stagnation of society has been to foster a sense of apprehension and diminished expectations for the future. If collective aspirations are no longer viable, then the scope for individual aspirations is also reduced. The contemporary preoccupation with the body is one consequence of this: if you cannot do much to change society or your place in it, at least you can mould your own body according to your own inclinations. The consequences of this narcissistic outlook range from the fads for body-building, tattooing and body-piercing to the increasing prevalence of morbid conditions of self-mutilation, anorexia and bulimia (Porter 1999). The intense social concern about health is closely related to the cult of the body: once you give up on any prospect of achieving progress in society, your horizons are reduced to securing your own physical survival:

> Investing in the body provides people with a means of self-expression and a way of potentially feeling good and increasing the control they have over their bodies. If one feels unable to exert control over an increasingly complex society, at least one can have some effect on the size, shape and appearance of one's body.
>
> (Shilling 1993: 7)

From this perspective, quantitative indicators of health (of the individual and of society) become more important than indicators of the quality of life. 'Life expectancy' – measured in units of time – becomes more important than any concern about how the additional time gained might be spent.

The dramatic increase in state intervention in the health-related behaviour of the individual over the past decade has taken place in parallel with the contraction of the traditional sphere of politics. The ending of the Cold War also brought to an end the polarities of left and right that had dominated parliamentary and electoral politics over the previous century. The unchallenged ascendancy of the capitalist system meant that debates about policy became superfluous and government was reduced to administration. Yet, conservative propagandists immediately felt the loss of their old adversaries and were now forced to find new ways of securing popular approval for a system which had an inescapable tendency to generate social instability and dissatisfaction. In this wider context, intervention in health served a number of purposes. By projecting an image of concern about issues of health and disease, the government hoped to bolster its flagging legitimacy. It also welcomed a mechanism for establishing more direct relations with citizens and thereby strengthening the authority of government over an increasingly fragmented society. Successive governments also sought to use these measures and more direct administrative reforms as means of securing tighter control over public expenditure on health.

When health becomes the goal of human endeavour it acquires an oppressive influence over the life of the individual. If people's lives are ruled by the measures they believe may help to prolong their existence, the quality of their lives is diminished. The tryanny of health means the ascendancy of the imperatives of biology over the aspirations of the human spirit. It provides the state, working both independently and through the agency of doctors and other health professionals, with a mechanism for extending its authority over the lives of each individual citizen and thereby over the whole of society.

Moving forward

How can we challenge the tyranny of health? Certainly not by clinging to tradition or by trying to return to that mythical golden age symbolised for many by the post-war NHS. It is not a question of going back, but of moving forward in a direction different from that charted by the current wave of reform. The first step is to clarify the specific features of our current predicament, in particular the links between, on the one hand, the tyranny of health and the crisis of medicine, and on the other, the stasis of the new world order that has come into being since the collapse of communism. A historical example may help to illuminate the distinctive character of the current moment.

The great nineteenth-century German pathologist Rudolph Virchow has become a heroic figure for the advocates of the new public health (Ashton, Seymour 1988: 91; Jacobson 1991: 107; Konner 1993: 71; Calman 1998: 172). His comment that 'medicine is a social science, and politics is nothing else but medicine on a large scale' is widely quoted and its spirit often invoked (Sigerist 1941: 93). But though this is a fine slogan, asserting with rhetorical flourish the common cause of medical practice and political struggle at a particular historical moment, Virchow's aphorism does not stand close inspection as an analysis of the relationship between medicine and society in general. Medicine is a clinical practice as well as being a social science: it must therefore, while recognising the importance of social factors in the causation of disease, give primacy to the needs of the individual. The primary concern of politics is with the needs of society as a whole, to which the concerns of the individual must be subordinate.

As well as pioneering the discipline of cellular pathology, Virchow was a lifelong political activist, a radical democratic deputy in the Reichstag and closely associated with liberal-left causes (Rosen 1993: 230–4). Two events in 1848 provided the context for his famous slogan: an epidemic of typhus in the impoverished district of Upper Silesia, which he was despatched to investigate as a junior member of a government commission, and the revolutionary upsurge against autocracy which shook Berlin, Paris and a number of other European cities, with which he strongly identified. In his (minority) report on the epidemic, Virchow emphasised the role of poverty, hunger, poor housing and sanitation in encouraging the spread of disease and advocated social reform as the most effective remedy. He argued that the best way to prevent a recurrence was to 'provide the inhabitants with efficient industry, improved agriculture, new roads, communal self-government, education, prosperity, liberty and democracy' (Evans 1987: 274). Virchow immediately identified the revolutionary democratic movements of 1848 – which were also hailed by Marx and Engels as the first manifestation of the potential of the emerging working class – as the social force that could effect the scale of reform required to prevent the epidemics raging in the squalor of rampant early capitalist development.

In the moment of 1848, Virchow's slogan linked the aspirations of radical doctors to tackle the social conditions of epidemic disease and the ambitions of the revolutionary movement to overthrow dictatorship. In the event, the revolutionary upsurge was contained and, as the regime in Prussia was consolidated under Bismarck in the latter part of the nineteenth century, Virchow became an increasingly isolated figure. Though in 1848 he had rejected the notion that epidemics resulted from some contagious factor, after Koch's discovery of the tubercle bacillus (the cause of tuberculosis) in 1884, he finally accepted the germ theory. However, he remained a staunch libertarian, strongly opposed to any concept of state control, maintaining that 'freedom from authoritarian government alone guaranteed freedom from infectious disease' (Evans 1987: 274).

In the Europe of the late 1980s, the movement for liberty and democracy that had emerged 150 years earlier finally collapsed. All aspirations for social progress through transcending the capitalist order, which had sustained generations of radicals from 1848 to 1968 and beyond, were now in abeyance. Indeed, not only were all prospects of social change through collective action now ruled out, the scope for individual initiative was also put in question. Doctors could now play a role in society, not in alliance with mass demo-cratic social movements, but only as agents of the state. This fundamental change in social context gives Virchow's slogan an entirely different meaning. In the absence of a forceful movement from below, medical intervention in society becomes a vehicle of government policy, not politics 'writ large', but politics on a small scale, petty, intrusive and moralising. Radical doctors may still project their desires for the redistribution of wealth to remove the social causes of health inequalities but, as the government's response confirms, its only interest is in improving social cohesion and stability. Hence doctors who take on a wider social role find themselves implementing policies which, far from offering greater liberty and democracy, have an inherently coercive character. What a bitter irony that Virchow, the great libertarian, now provides an aura of radical legitimacy for an authoritarian government health policy.

The pre-eminent role of health in Western society since the early 1990s is linked to a significant shift in the boundaries between the spheres of public and personal life, and to changes in the relation-ship between the state and the medical profession. Challenging the tyranny of health in the context of the wider social changes we have discussed, involves redefining these boundaries. This means, on the one hand, defending the autonomy of the medical profession and, on the other, upholding the autonomy of the patient. Let's take these in turn.

Professional autonomy

In his celebrated sociological study of medical professionalism, Eliot Freidson emphasised that 'the only truly important and uniform criterion for distinguishing professions from other occupations is the fact of autonomy – a position of legitimate control over work' (Freidson 1970: 82). He further argued that professional autonomy was 'the critical outcome of the interaction between political and economic power and occupational representation, interaction sometimes facilitated by educational institutions and other devices which successfully persuade the state that the occupation's work is reliable and valuable' (Freidson 1970: 82–3). The licensing system introduced in Britain by the 1858 Medical Act sought to guarantee the public that a registered doctor was a 'safe general practitioner' and the GMC policed both the conduct of doctors with their patients and in their relations with other practitioners. It also allowed a unified profession to project an ethical orientation which put public service before self interest. As Freidson put it, 'the profession's service orientation is a public imputation it has successfully won in a process by which its leaders have persuaded society to grant and support its autonomy' (Freidson 1970: 82). In the course of its development from the foundations established in the 1850s, the medical profession had to negotiate two key sets of relationships – with the state and with the market.

Doctors were always ambivalent about the state, an ambivalence that persisted despite the advance of state intervention in health from the late nineteenth century onwards. On the one hand, doctors recognised that state patronage was crucial to the establishment and maintenance of their professional hegemony. On the other, they regarded state incursions as a threat to cherished traditions of individual freedom and professional autonomy.

While doctors recognised the necessity for state sponsorship, they remained jealous of their professional independence, particularly emphasising the threat of external interference to the integrity of the confidential doctor–patient relationship. Hence, while generally welcoming a state licensing system, the medical profession ensured that this system was administered by a General Medical Council dominated by representatives of the profession itself. Thus was inaugurated the principle of self-regulation, albeit within a state-imposed framework, a principle vigorously upheld by the profession and respected by the state. In 1975, for example, an independent commission set up to review the GMC, unequivocally endorsed self-regulation: 'It is the essence of a professional skill that it deals with matters unfamiliar to the layman, and it follows that only those in the profession are in a position to judge many of the matters of standards of professional conduct which will be involved' (Merrison 1975: 133).

Though in their posture of resistance to the state, doctors have often claimed an ideological affinity for the principles of the free market, in reality their relations with the world of commerce are also characterised by a high degree of ambivalence. In his survey of the medical profession in the USA, where entrepreneurial principles are most fervently cherished – not least among doctors – Paul Starr noted that 'the contradiction between professionalism and the rule of the market is long-standing and unavoidable' (Starr 1982: 23). Traditional physicians regarded the market as a threat to both income and status, as they were forced to compete with diverse unscrupulous practitioners and also deal with attempts to turn them into mere employees. In response, doctors – in common with other aspiring professionals – tried to distinguish themselves from tradesmen and businessmen by claiming a commitment to a higher cause than vulgar commercial interests: 'In justifying the public's trust, professionals have set higher standards of conduct for themselves than the minimal rules governing the marketplace and maintained that they can be judged under those standards only by each other, not by laymen' (Starr 1982: 23). Whereas the market ideal is that the consumer rules, the ideal of a profession 'calls for the sovereignty of its members' independent, authoritative judgement'. From this perspective, a quack is a practitioner who tries to please his customers rather than his colleagues. Professional organisation is a form of resistance to the market, which seeks to restrict competition by regulating the supply of medical services, though, paradoxically, a degree of independence from the market was only achieved through increasing dependence on the state.

The conception of the 'competent general practitioner' is very important in the traditions of the medical profession. Once registered as such with the GMC, doctors were independent professionals who could put up their own plate and practise medicine according to their own judgements and aspirations. The notion that professional excellence could be guaranteed by some external agency, such as the state, was alien to the medical profession in its ascendant phase. Professional autonomy has long been recognised as vital to the integrity of the doctor–patient relationship. This is, ideally, an intimate relationship, developed in the course of repeated interaction, often in the context of critical life events – birth, serious illness, death. It is a personal relationship between two idiosyncratic individuals, significant to both and, when successful, mutually rewarding as well as being beneficial to the patient. Inevitably, as in all relationships, reality sometimes lags some distance behind the ideal, yet there has always been enough of a glimpse of the ideal for both doctor and patient to aspire to achieve it. Like all intimate relationships, this one is inscrutable to the outsider – and also often, to some degree, to the participants.

In the past the GMC was mainly concerned with 'bad' doctors. It investigated allegations of malpractice or other misdemeanours, and if such charges were upheld, doctors could be struck off the medical register. But, just as public confidence in the medical profession was little affected by periodic scandals concerning corrupt or lecherous doctors, neither did it depend on the vigorous pursuit of such rogues by the GMC. The prestige of the medical profession, had quite different – and until the last decade, quite secure – foundations in the successes of scientific medicine and the vitality of the doctor–patient relationship. While the GMC policed a delinquent fringe of practitioners, the mediocrity of many doctors was tacitly accepted as a price worth paying for the overall benefits of an independent profession. The key change of the 1990s is that long-tolerated variations in styles and standards of medical practice have suddenly been judged to be 'unacceptable'. This judgement was made, at least in the first instance, not by the public or by the media, but by doctors themselves. One of the ironies of this shift is that it has taken place after a period of dramatic improvements in standards.

One of the key demands of reformers, from both inside and outside the medical profession, is for an increase in the proportion of non-medical, lay members on the GMC. In the aftermath of the Shipman case, more radical critics of the GMC proposed that it should have a lay majority, thus effectively bringing professional self-regulation to an end. Lay members were first introduced onto the GMC in 1950 and their numbers have increased substantially in recent years. Though reformers seem to assume that lay members provide some sort of representation of the public, the mode of selection – by appointment by the Privy Council – means that they are more an instrument of state control than a mechanism of democratic accountability. Leading figures in the RCGP assert that the 'input of lay people is critical to ensure coverage of areas to do with communication and attitudes to patients' (Southgate, Pringle 1999). Yet they do not explain why lay people should be better judges of these matters than doctors who have both professional and personal experience of doctor–patient interactions. Nor do they indicate the nature and scale of the lay input, or how such people would be selected, trained or paid. Following the pattern of such appointments to diverse quangos, they could be expected to be selected according to their loyalty to New Labour and its leadership. The willingness of doctors to concede the right to judge their fitness to practise to those who include such cronies and toadies reflects an alarming loss of professional self-respect.

The independent general practitioner, competent on qualification, symbolised the confidence of the medical profession in the nineteenth century. By contrast, the 'never quite competent' GP, one who requires continuous formal instruction and regulation, mentoring and monitoring, support and counselling, symbolises the abject state of the profession at the start of the new millennium. But, while some GPs are drawn into the process of assessing their colleagues' fitness and many more are continuously collecting evidence to justify their fitness to practise, who will see the patients? And what will patients think of doctors who have so little faith in themselves that they put their trust in formal procedures of assessment and regulation? Far from restoring public confidence in medicine, the proposed system of revalidation is destined to damage it still further.

The immediate response to any criticism of the drive to revalidation is the demand for a superior alternative. But revalidation is the answer to the wrong question: it is not a matter of proposing an alternative response, but of reposing the question – what is the real problem of contemporary medicine? It is not underperforming and unacceptable GPs or inadequate regulatory procedures – these are old and familiar problems. The real problem lies with the style of practice deemed excellent by the leaders of the profession, a style which is destined to be promoted still further by the revalidation procedures. This approach is characterised by a shift of medical practice away from the care and treatment of patients towards the regulation of behaviour and the rationing of resources. It results in individual GPs devoting less time to their own patients and spending more time in activities remote from the patients. It also has the effect of making doctor–patient relations more conflictual and instrumental, as doctors try to persuade their patients to adopt healthy lifestyles and undergo screening tests (partly in the cause of making targets) and patients see doctors as the front line of the government's drive to curtail NHS spending on drugs and hospital treatment.

If doctors are concerned about restoring public trust, we should first recall what created public trust in the medical profession in the first place. This should lead to a renewed commitment to medical science and a determination to defend it against the anti-scientific prejudices which have recently become influential, not only in society as a whole, but more damagingly within medicine itself. It should also lead to a recognition of the importance of sustaining the personal doctor–patient relationship which has always been the bedrock of general practice, but is threatened by recent bureaucratic trends, not least by the drive towards revalidation.

The autonomy of the patient

According to GP philosopher Peter Toon, 'autonomy has become a buzzword in medical ethics' (Toon 1999: 16). This concept 'has been at the centre of the attack led by a recent generation of non-physician medical ethicists and patient representatives on the arrogance of medical paternalism'. But this narrow focus on doctors as the major threat to the autonomy of the patient underestimates both the impact of wider social and political forces on the doctor–patient relationship and the potential for doctors and patients to work together to combat the oppressive consequences of these influences.

We have considered two interlinked trends which have the effect of diminishing individual autonomy: the medicalisation of life and the politicisation of medicine. The first involves the proliferation of categories of disease to cover wider and wider areas of human experience and a growing proportion of the population. It also involves extending medical jurisdiction over diverse areas of personal and social life in the cause of preventing disease. The identification of more and more people deemed to be exhibiting some form of chemical dependency or psychological deficiency is another feature of medicalisation. By exaggerating disability and incapacity, this boom in diagnostic activity degrades individual autonomy and justifies professional intervention in personal life on a growing scale. Though the shift of doctors away from a focus on the individual patient towards a wider social and political role is often presented as a progressive development motivated by concerns to tackle the effects of poverty and discrimination, as we have seen, it tends to result in intrusive and coercive measures. Collaboration between doctors and agencies such as the police, local authority social services, and voluntary organisations such as the National Society for the Prevention of Cruelty to Children, inevitably draws doctors into a more authoritarian role. The incorporation of medical representatives into bodies, such as primary care groups and primary care trusts, responsible for allocating – and rationing – resources pushes doctors into containing patient demands for health care while protecting politicians from the resulting public hostility (Heath 1995: 44).

The changing role of the doctor also changes the role of the patient, who has increasingly become the object of medical intervention rather than the subject seeking medical care or treatment. From the new public health perspective, any consultation between doctor and patient is an opportunity for health promotion and disease prevention, for raising awareness of whatever condition is currently fashionable – or for explaining to the patient that their expectations must be reconciled with priorities as dictated by the government and enforced through guidelines and waiting lists. Doctors are constantly advised to take advantage of any encounter with patients to ask about smoking and drinking, diet and exercise (and to record the answers) and to follow up with the appropriate exhortations. Like Iona Heath, 'I believe that all my patients are fully informed of the dangers of smoking' – being advised that cigarettes are bad for their health when they come in to the surgery with bronchitis (or something worse) simply compounds their demoralisation (Heath 1995: 11). Inquiries in such circumstances into whether they are also currently experiencing domestic violence or are engaging consistently in the practices of safe sex are unwarranted (and prurient) intrusions into personal life.

The threat to patient autonomy from 'opportunist' screening is being increasingly recognised. Given the way that target payments have led GPs to recommend cervical smears to women who come in to the surgery for some other purpose, Toon asks 'whether taking the opportunity provided by a patient's consultation to deal with an issue on the doctor's but not the patient's agenda is an infringement of the patient's autonomy' (Toon 1994: 34). He rightly condemns incentive policies which lead to inappropriate pressures on patients to submit to screening procedures – and even to the removal of recalcitrant patients from GP lists – as treating people as 'ends not means' and as being 'in conflict with fundamental respect for persons' (Toon 1999: 30). However his attempt to resolve this conflict by distinguishing between 'offering, as opposed to imposing' screening procedures is unsatisfactory. The immediate problem is that, as the screening authorities recognise, a fully informed patient may be less likely to consent to procedures such as smears and mammograms. The more fundamental problem is the presumption that offering patients information can have the effect of 'empowering them to make more informed choices' (Toon 1999: 31). Given the context that, in our society, the GP stands in a position of considerable social authority in relation to the vast majority of patients, 'offering information' cannot be considered as neutral interaction between equal individuals. This is particularly the case if the patient is consulting the GP in relation to some illness and is feeling rather vulnerable, and even more so in the situation where the GP has telephoned the patient at home to indicate that a smear test is overdue. Most women would experience such an offer as one that was difficult to refuse and, as such, it has the effect of reinforcing medical power rather than transferring it to the patient.

The transformation of medical practice has provoked increasing tension and conflict in relations between doctors and patients. From the doctors' side, a glance at the popular weekly GP news magazines reveals a preoccupation with violence from patients, with regular accounts of assaults, details of training in self-defence and security procedures and accounts of special arrangements between surgeries and the police. This preoccupation is extraordinary because, in my experience in an area with a high level of violent crime, such incidents are as rare as they have ever been; what has changed is the fact they are perceived as manifestations of a universal threat rather than as occasional bizarre events. (It is striking that similar concerns can be found in the magazines of teachers, social workers, indeed in all occupations in contact with the public.) Another recurrent theme in the GP press (and that of other professions) is that of the unprecedented levels of stress in the job, resulting, at least in part, from the excessive demands of patients, with warnings of the dangers of 'burn-out' or breakdown, unless doctors seek appropriate counselling and support. From the patients' side, the decline of deference is proclaimed by numerous self-help groups and by the growing scale of complaints (encouraged by the proliferation of complaints procedures) and, most importantly, by the dramatic increase in litigation (though most claims are settled out of court). Once distinguished by their confidence and composure, doctors now often seem to regard their patients with fear and rage; many of their once acquiescent patients now view their doctors with undisguised suspicion and hostility.

In response to recent trends in doctor–patient relations, medical ethicists and other self-appointed patient representatives have welcomed measures to extend official regulation of the medical profession and to make available more information about medical performance, in the form of hospital league tables and other indicators. Such procedures are regarded as providing greater openness and accountability, as challenging medical paternalism and empowering patients. But it is impossible to resolve the mismatch in knowledge and expertise between doctor and patient at the level of the individual encounter. This is particularly the case when the patient's relative ignorance is compounded by the incapacity resulting from illness and decisions need to be taken promptly. Even when the gulf between doctor and patient can be reduced by recourse to league tables and the internet, a leap of faith is still required. This leap of faith in the medical consultation assumes a level of trust, not only between the individual doctor and patient, but between the medical profession and the public, and within society as a whole. Whereas trust is likely to be damaged still further by the intervention of third parties, its best safeguard remains the relationship between the individual doctor and individual patient – if it is strictly confined to medical matters.

Redrawing the boundaries

Overturning the tyranny of health involves challenging both the medicalisation of life and the politicisation of medicine. At a time when the subordination of the medical profession to the state has become a strategic device for pushing forward the agenda of medicalisation and for securing the government's short-term political objectives, the autonomy of the profession offers some safeguards for both doctors and the public. Despite the undoubted abuses of professional authority by doctors, past and present, the principles of self-regulation still provide a defence against state interference – a much more potent source of abuses. Given current moves towards more authoritarian government, any focus of independence offers a potential for resistance to tyrannical trends.

The erosion of the boundaries between the public and the private spheres is one of the most ominous trends in modern society, and one in which doctors, with their unique access to the intimate aspects of personal life, play an important role. The declining status of public institutions and of public life in general has encouraged a retreat into the private realm – at a time when the private realm has itself been opened up to public scrutiny to an unprecedented degree. With their recommendations for changes in lifestyle and their invitations to screening, and their guidelines on tackling domestic violence, sexual abuse, defective parenting and numerous other social evils, doctors are at the cutting edge of the drive to extend professional regulation over personal life. The other side of this coin is the projection of private passions into the public realm as manifested in the elevation of emotion over reason in political debate and the outpouring of ersatz grief in response to events such as the death of Princess Diana in 1997.

The particular difficulty of proposing a clarification of the line between the public and the private is that, not only is there little apparent resistance to the relaxation of this boundary, but these trends are widely celebrated. New Labour politicians welcome the contribution of greater 'emotional literacy' to public life, while campaigning doctors regard the opening up of the private sphere as a positive step towards exposing the dark secrets of the family and its abusive and exploitative relationships. There is little recognition that promoting the legitimacy of 'feelings' as an alternative to political argument, risks 'eradicating altogether altogether a prime requisite of politics – the need for judgement based on criteria which are public in nature' (Elshtain 1997). Nor is there much concern about the danger of diminishing the personal sphere, even though this closes down the space of personal development in intimate relationships and ultimately weakens individual autonomy. However, the consequences of blurring the distinction between the public and the private are grave: the replacement of political accountability with sentimentality (as, for example, in Tony Blair's 'trust me' plea that the government's decision to exempt motor racing from the ban on cigarette sponsorship in 1997 had not been influenced by Bernie Ecclestone's donation to the Labour Party) and the degradation of subjectivity.

In response, we should seek neither to glorify nor disparage either the public or the private realms in themselves, but to insist on the importance of maintaining the distinction. Doctors can make a useful contribution by restraining the tendency for medical practice to expand into more and more areas of personal and social life. This means redefining medicine in terms of treating the sick and leaving the well alone. Given both the lack of a strong scientific justification for much of the work of health promotion and the authoritarian dynamic that such activity inevitably acquires in the current political climate, there is a strong case for abandoning it. Doctors should stop trying to moralise their patients and concentrate on treating them:

> In the words of a wise physician, it is part of the doctor's function to make it possible for his patients to go on doing the pleasant things that are bad for them – smoking too much, eating too much, drinking too much – without killing themselves any sooner than is necessary.
>
> (Dubos 1960: 171)

Proposing a much more restricted definition of medical practice does not mean that doctors should ignore the social determinants of illness and disease. It means distinguishing clearly between taking up these issues in a political and in a medical way. In the current climate any attempt to pursue political issues through medical practice is likely to have adverse consequences for patients, for doctors and for the doctor–patient relationship. In these circumstances, the first responsiblity of a doctor *as a doctor* is to provide medical treatment for individual patients. Doctors who aspire to a wider political role would be best advised to pursue this, not in their surgery, but in the public sphere, where issues of patient and professional autonomy should have the highest priority. If the medical profession cannot defend its own integrity against government interference it is unlikely to make much headway in challenging the social causes of ill health. If doctors cannot take a stand against schemes of state-sponsored, medically-sanctioned coercion, then they risk finding themselves incapable of maintaining any sort of therapeutic relationship with their patients.

BIBLIOGRAPHY

Abbasi, K. (1999) 'Butchers and gropers', *BMJ*, 317: 1600–01.

Acheson, D. (1988) *Public Health in England: The Report of the Committee of Inquiry into the Future Development of the Public Health Function*, Cm 289, London: HMSO.

Action on Addiction (1997) Press pack, October. London: Action on Addiction.

Advisory Committee to the Surgeon-General of the Public Health Service (1964) *Smoking and Health*, Atlanta: US Department of Health, Education and Welfare.

Advisory Council on the Misuse of Drugs (1982) *Treatment and Rehabilitation*, London: HMSO.

——(1984) *Guidelines on Good Clinical Practice in the Treatment of Drug Misuse*, London: HMSO.

Allen, I. (1994) *Doctors and their Careers*, London: Policy Studies Institute.

American Psychiatric Association (1994) *Diagnostic and Statistical Manual of Mental Disorders*, fourth edition (DSM IV), Washington DC: APA.

Anderson, C.M. (1999) 'Smear tests were not on trial but should have been', *BMJ*, 318: 1007.

Anderson, D. (1994) 'The health activists: educators or propagandists?' in *Health, Lifestyle and Environment*, London/New York: Social Affairs Unit/Manhattan Institute.

Armstrong, D. (1986) 'The invention of infant mortality', *Sociology of Health and Illness*, 8: 3: 211–32 (September).

Ashton, J., Seymour, H. (eds) (1988) *The New Public Health*, Milton Keynes/Philadelphia: Open University Press.

Austoker, J. (1994a) 'Cancer prevention in primary care: screening and self-examination for breast cancer', *BMJ*, 309: 168–74.

——(1994b) 'Cancer prevention in primary care: screening for ovarian, prostatic and testicular cancer', *BMJ*, 309: 315–20.

Baum, M. (1995) 'Screening for breast cancer, time to think – and stop', *Lancet*, 346: 436–7.

Beck, U. (1992) *The Risk Society*, London: Sage.

174

Benzeval, M., Donald, A. (1999) 'The role of the NHS in tackling inequalities in health' in D. Gordon *et al.* (eds) *Inequalities in Health*, Bristol: Policy Press.

Benzeval, M., Judge, K., Whitehead, M. (eds) (1995) *Tackling Inequalities in Health*, London: Kings Fund.

Beral, V., Hermon, C., Reeves, G., Peto, R. (1995) 'Sudden fall in breast cancer rates in England and Wales', *Lancet*, 345: 1642–3.

Berger, J., Mohr, J. (1967) *A Fortunate Man*, London: Allen Lane.

Berger, P. (1994) 'Towards a religion of health activism' in *Health, Lifestyle and Environment*, London/New York: Social Affairs Unit/Manhattan Institute.

Berridge, V. (1979) 'Morality and medical science: concepts of narcotic addiction in Britain', *Annals of Science*, 36: 67–85.

——(1998) 'Science and policy: the case of post-war British smoking policy' in S. Lock *et al.* (eds) *Ashes to Ashes*, Amsterdam/Atlanta: Rodopi.

——(1999) *Opium and the People* (revised edition), London: Free Association.

Bewley, S., Friend, J., Mezey, G. (eds) (1997) *Violence against Women*, London: Royal College of Obstetrics and Gynaecology.

Binchy, J.M., Molyneux, E.M., Manning, J. (1994) 'Accidental ingestion of methadone by children in Merseyside', *BMJ*, 308: 1335–6.

Black Report (1980) *Inequalities of Health*, Report of a Research Working Group, Chairman Sir Douglas Black, London: DHSS (subsequently published as *The Black Report* (1982), London: Pelican.

Bloor, K., Maynard, M. (1998) *Clinical Governance: Clinician Heal Thyself?*, London: Institute of Health Services Management.

BMA (1986) *Alternative Therapy*, London: BMA.

——(1990) *The BMA Guide to Living With Risk*, London: Penguin.

——(1993) *Complementary Medicine: New Approach to Good Practice*, London: BMA.

——(1995) *Inequality and Health*, London: BMA.

——(1997) *The Misuse of Drugs*, London: BMA.

——(1998) *Health and Environmental Impact Assessment*, London: BMA/Earthscan.

——(1998) *Domestic Violence: a health care issue?*, London: BMA.

——(January 1999) 'Public trust in doctors remains high', Press Release, London: BMA.

——(1999) *The Impact of Genetic Modification on Agriculture, Food and Health*, London: BMA.

Bonneux, L., Barendregt, J.J. (1994) 'Ischaemic heart disease and cholesterol', *BMJ*, 308: 1038.

Bookchin, M. (1995) *Re-enchanting Humanity*, London: Cassell.

Booth, C. (1998) 'Smoking and the Royal College of Physicians' in S. Lock *et al.* (eds) *Ashes to Ashes*, Amsterdam/Atlanta: Rodopi.

Boston Women's Health Collective (1972) *Our Bodies Ourselves*, Boston: Boston Women's Health Collective.

Bradley, A. (1999) 'Another HIV negative', *LM Magazine*, October: 36–7.

Brandt, A. (1998) 'Blow some my way: passive smoking, risk and American culture' in S. Lock *et al.* (eds) *Ashes to Ashes*, Amsterdam/Atlanta: Rodopi.

Brandt, A.M. (1997) 'Behaviour, disease and health in the twentieth century USA', in A.M. Brandt and P. Rozin (eds) *Morality and Health*, London: Routledge.

Buckley, G. (1999) 'Revalidation is the answer', *BMJ*, 319: 1145–6.

Buckman, R. (1994) *How to Break Bad News*, Toronto: Pan.

Bunker, J.P., Houghton, J., Baum, M. (1998) 'Putting the risk of breast cancer in perspective', *BMJ*, 317: 1307–09.

Burnet, M. (1971) *Genes, Dreams and Realities*, Aylesbury, Bucks: Medical and Technical.

Bynum, W.F. (1994) *Science and the Practice of Medicine in the Nineteenth Century*, Cambridge: Cambridge University Press.

Cairns, A., Roberts, I.S.D., Benbow, E.W. (1996) 'Characteristics of fatal methadone overdose in Manchester, 1985–94', *BMJ*, 313: 264–5.

California Environmental Protection Agency (1997) *Health Effects of Exposure to Environmental Tobacco Smoke*, Sacramento: California EPA.

Calman, K. (1998) *The Potential for Health*, Oxford: Oxford University Press.

Charlton, B. (1994) 'Health promotion and NHS reform: A critique of *Health of the Nation*' in J. LeFanu (ed.) *Preventionitis: The Exaggerated Claims of Health Promotion*, London: Social Affairs Unit.

——(1995) 'A critique of Geoffrey Rose's "population strategy" for preventive medicine', *Journal of the Royal Society of Medicine*, 88: 607–10.

Clark, A. (1994) *Diaries*, London: Phoenix.

Cleare, A.J., Wessely, S.C. (1997) 'Just what the doctor ordered – more alcohol and sex', *BMJ*, 315: 1637–8.

Cochrane, A. (1972) *Effectiveness and Efficiency: random reflections on health services*, London: Nuffield Provincial Hospitals Trust.

——(1976) 'Some reflections' in G. McLachlan (ed.) *A Question of Quality: Roads to Assurance in Medical Care,* London: Nuffield Provincial Hospitals Trust / Oxford University Press.

Cochrane, A.L., Holland, W.W. (1971) 'Validation of screening procedures', *BMJ*, 27:3–8.

COMA (Committee on Medical Aspects of Food Policy) (1994) *Nutritional Aspects of Cardiovascular Disease*, London: HMSO.

Commission on Social Justice (1994) *Social Justice*, London: Vintage.

Copas, J.B., Shi, J.Q. (2000) 'Reanalysis of epidemiological evidence on lung cancer and passive smoking', *BMJ*, 320: 417–18.

BIBLIOGRAPHY

Craft, W. (1994) 'WHO denounces health benefits of alcohol', *BMJ*, 309: 1242.

Crawford, R. (1977) 'You are dangerous to your health: the ideology and politics of victim-blaming', *International Journal of Health Services*, 7 (4) 663–680.

Curtis, H., Hoolaghan, T., Jewitt, C. (eds) (1995) *Sexual Health Promotion in General Practice*, Oxford/New York: Radcliffe Medical Press.

Dalrymple, T. (1998) *Mass Listeria*, London: Andre Deutsch.

Dargie, H., Grant, S. (1992) 'The role of exercise' in *The Health of the Nation: the BMJ View*, London: *BMJ*.

Davey, B., Gray, A., Seale, C. (1984) *Health and Disease*, Buckingham/Philadelphia: Open University Press.

Davies, H.T.O., Mannion, R. (1999) *Clinical Governance: Striking a Balance Between Checking and Trusting*, York: Centre for Health Economics.

Day, P., Klein, R. (1990) *Inspecting the Inspectorates*, London: Joseph Rowntree Foundation.

Dent, J.A. (1993) 'Students like new curriculum', *BMJ*, 306: 1410 (22 May).

Department of Health (1979) *Eating for Health*, London: HMSO.

——(1988) *Short-Term Prediction of HIV Infection and Aids in England and Wales* (Cox Report), London: HMSO.

——(1989) *Working for Patients*, Cmnd 555, London: HMSO.

——(1991) *While You Are Pregnant*, London: HMSO.

——(1991) *The Health of the Nation*, Consultative Document, Cmnd 1523, London: HMSO.

——(1992) *The Health of the Nation*, London: HMSO (Cmnd 1986).

——(1995) *Sensible Drinking*, London: DoH.

——(1997) *The New NHS: Modern. Dependable*, London: HMSO.

——(1997) *On the State of the Public Health: The Annual Report of the Chief Medical Officer of the Department of Health for the Year 1996*, London: HMSO.

——(1998a) *A First Class Service: Quality in the New NHS*, London: Stationery Office.

——(1998b) *The National Survey of NHS Patients: General Practice*, London: Stationery Office.

——(February 1998) *Our Healthier Nation: A Contract for Health* (Green Paper), London: Stationery Office.

——(1999) *Drug Misuse and Dependence: Guidelines on Clinical Management*, London: Stationery Office.

——(July 1999) *Saving Lives: Our Healthier Nation* (White Paper), London: Stationery Office.

——(November 1999) *Supporting Doctors, Protecting Patients*, London: DoH.

Department of Health and Social Security (1976) *Prevention and Health: Everybody's Business*, Discussion document, London: HMSO.

——(1977) *Prevention and Health: Everybody's Business*, Cmnd 7047, London: HMSO.

Doll, R. (1998) 'The first reports of smoking and lung cancer', in S. Lock *et al.* (eds) *Ashes to Ashes*, Amsterdam/Atlanta: Rodopi.

Doll, R., Peto, R., Hall, E., Wheatley, W., Gray, R. (1994) 'Mortality in relation to alchol consumption', *BMJ*: 309: 911–18.

Dollery, C. (1978) *The End of an Age of Optimism*, Oxford: Nuffield Provincial Hospitals Trust.

Dubos, R. (1960) *The Mirage of Health*, London: Allen & Unwin.

Dunnigan, M. (1993) 'The problem with cholesterol', *BMJ*, 306: 1355–6.

Durodie, B. (1999) *Poisonous Dummies*, Cambridge: European Science and Environment Forum.

Ebrahim, S., Bennet, R. (2000) 'Health promotion activity should be retargeted at secondary prevention', *BMJ*, 320: 185.

Ebrahim, S., Davey Smith, G. (1997) 'Systematic review of randomised controlled trials of multiple risk factor interventions for preventing coronary heart disease', *BMJ*, 314: 1666–73.

Ehrenreich, B., English, D. (1974) *Witches, Midwives and Nurses*, London: Compendium.

Elshtain, J.B. (1997) 'The Displacement of Politics' in J. Weintraub and K. Kumar (eds) *Public and Private in Thought and Practice: Perspectives on a Grand Dichotomy*, Chicago: University of Chicago Press.

Emery, J.L., Waite, J.A. (2000) 'These deaths must be prevented without victimising parents', *BMJ*: 320: 310.

Evans, R.J. (1987) *Death in Hamburg*, London: Penguin.

Farrant, W. (1991) 'Addressing the contradictions: health promotion and community health action in the UK', *International Journal of Health Services*, 21; 3: 423–9.

Farrant, W., Russell, J. (1986) *The Politics of Health Information*, London: Institute of Education.

Fielding, H. (1997) *Bridget Jones' Diary*, London: Picador.

Fitzpatrick, M. (1998) 'How now mad cow?' in I. McCalman, B. Penny, M. Cook (eds) *Mad Cows and Modernity*, Canberra: Australian National University.

——(1998) 'No backbone in beef crisis', *LM Magazine*, February: 32–4.

——Fitzpatrick, M. (1999) 'Should parenting be taught?', *Guardian*, 4 December.

Fitzpatrick, M., Hehir, B. (1999) 'The dangers of safe sun', *LM Magazine*, July/August: 10–11.

Fitzpatrick, M., Milligan, D. (1987) *The Truth About The Aids Panic*, London: Junius.

Fletcher, R.H., Fletcher, S.W. (1990) 'Clinical practice guidelines', *Annals of Internal Medicine*, 113: 645–6.

Flexner, A. (1910) *Medical Education in the United States and Canada*, New York: Carnegie Foundation.

——(1925) *Medical Education*, New York: Macmillan.

Foucault, M. (1961) *Madness and Civilisation*, London: Tavistock.

——(1979) *The History of Sexuality*, London: Penguin.

Freidson, E. (1970) *Profession of Medicine*, New York: Dodd Mead.

Fukuyama, F. (1989) 'The end of history', *National Interest*, 16.

Furedi, A. (1999) 'The public health implications of the 1995 "pill scare"', *Human Reproduction Update*, 5 (6): 621–6.

Furedi, F. (1992) *Mythical Past, Elusive Future*, London: Pluto.

——(1997) *Culture of Fear*, London: Cassell.

——(2000) *Parent Scaring: What Can We Do About Paranoid Parenting?*, London: Penguin.

—— (forthcoming) *State of Emotion*.

General Medical Council (1993) *Tomorrow's Doctors*, London: GMC.

Giddens, A. (1994) *Beyond Left and Right*, Cambridge: Polity.

——(1999) 'Why the old left is wrong on equality', *New Statesman*, 25 October.

Gillott, J., Kumar, M. (1995) *Science and the Retreat from Reason*, London: Merlin.

Glossop, M., Marsden, J., Stewart, D., Lehmann, P., Strang, J. (1999) 'Methadone treatment practices and outcome for opiate addicts treated in drug clincs and in general practice', *British Journal of General Practice*, 49: 31–4.

Goffman, E. (1961) *Asylums*, New York: Anchor, Doubleday (1974 edn, Penguin).

Goodhart, C., Layzell, S., Cook, A., Graffy, J. (1999) 'Family support in general practice', *Journal of the Royal Society of Medicine*, 92: 525–8.

Goodman, N.W. (1998) 'Clinical governance', *BMJ*, 317: 1725–7.

Gostin, L. (1997) 'The legal regulation of smoking (and smoking): public health or secular morality', in A.M. Brandt and P. Rozin (eds) *Morality and Health*, London: Routledge.

Gotzsche, P.C., Olsen, O. (2000) 'Is screening for breast cancer with mammography justifiable?', *Lancet*, 355: 129–34.

Graham, H. (1987) 'Women's smoking and family health', *Social Science and Medicine*, 25: 47–56.

——(1994) 'Gender and class as dimensions of smoking behaviour in Britain – insights from a study of mothers', *Social Science and Medicine*, 38: 691–8.

Grant, L. (1993) *Sexing the Millennium*, London: HarperCollins.

Gray, A.(1993) *World Health and Disease*, Buckingham: Open University Press.

Green, M.A. (1999) 'Time to put "cot death" to bed?', *BMJ*, 319: 697–700.

Greenwood, J., Zealley, H., Gorman, D., Fineron, P., Squires, T. (1997) 'Deaths related to methadone have doubled in Lothian', *BMJ*, 314: 1763.

Hackshaw, A.K., Law, M.R., Wald, N.J. (1997) 'The accumulated evidence on lung cancer and environmental tobacco smoke', *BMJ*, 315: 980–8.

Halsey, A.H. (ed.) (1988) *British Social Trends Since 1900*, London: Macmillan.

Harkin, K., Quinn, C., Bradley, F. (1999) 'Storing methadone in babies' bottles puts young children at risk', *BMJ*, 318: 329–30.

Harland, J., White, M., Drinkwater, C., Chinn, D., Farr, L., Howel, D. (1999) 'The Newcastle exercise project: a randomised controlled trial of methods to promote physical activity in primary care', *BMJ*, 319: 828–32.

Harris, M. (1994) *Magic in the Surgery*, London: Social Affairs Unit.

Heath, I. (1995) *The Mystery of General Practice*, London: Nuffield Provincial Hospitals Trust.

——(1995) 'Commentary: the perils of checklist medicine', *BMJ*, 311: 373.

——(1999) *Domestic violence: the general practitioner's role,* London: Royal College of General Practitioners.

Home Office, Department of Health, Department of Education and Science, Welsh Office (1991) *Working Together*, London: HMSO.

Horton, R. (1998) 'Yesterday's doctors', *Lancet*, 352: 1566–67.

Hunter, D. (1994) 'From tribalism to corporatism: the managerial challenge to medical dominance' in J. Gabe, D. Kelleher, G. Williams (eds) *Challenging Medicine*, London: Routledge.

Iliffe, S., Tai, S.S., Gould, M., Thorogood, M., Hillsdon, M. (1994) 'Prescribing exercise in general practice', *BMJ*, 309: 494–5.

Illich, I. (1975) *Medical Nemesis*, London: Calder & Boyars.

Inglis, B. (1981) *The Diseases of Civilisation*, London: Hodder and Stoughton.

Jackson, P. (1995) 'Passive smoking' in R. Bunton, S. Nettleton, R. Burrows (eds) *The Sociology of Health Promotion*, London: Routledge.

Jackson, R., Feder, G. (1998) 'Guidelines for clinical guidelines', *BMJ*, 317: 427–8.

James, O. (1997) *Britain on the Couch*, London: Century.

Jellinek, E.M. (1960) *The disease concept of alcoholism*, New Haven, Connecticut: Hill House Press.

Jewell, T. (1993) 'Counselling in general practice', *BMJ*, 306: 390.

Johnstone, J.R. (1991) 'Scientific fact or scientific delusion' in *Health, Lifestyle and the Environment*, London: Social Affairs Unit/Manhattan Institute.

Karpf, A. (1988) *Doctoring the Media*, London: Routledge.

Keen, J. (1999) 'Managing drug misuse in general practice', *BMJ*, 318: 1503–04.

Keen, J., Rowse, G., Mathers, N., Campbell, M., Seivewright, N. (2000) 'Can methadone maintenance for heroin-dependent patients retained in general practice reduce criminal conviction rates and time spent in prison?', *British Journal of General Practice*, 50: 48–9.

Kennedy, I. (1981) *The Unmasking of Medicine*, London: Allen & Unwin.

Knowles, J.H. (1977) 'The Responsibility of the Individual', *Daedalus*, 106: 57–80.

Konner, M. (1993) *The Trouble with Medicine*, London: BBC.

Kramer, P. (1994) *Listening to Prozac*, London: Fourth Estate.

Kristol, I. (1994) 'The good life and the new class' in *Health, Lifestyle and the Environment*, London/New York: Social Affairs Unit/Manahattan Institute.

Laing, R.D. (1960) *The Divided Self*, London: Tavistock (Penguin 1965).

Lalonde, M. (1974) *A New Perspective on the Health of Canadians*, Ottawa: Ministry of Supply and Services.

Lang, T. (1998) 'BSE and CJD: recent developments', in S. Ratzan (ed.), *The Mad Cow Crisis*, London: UCL Press.

Law, M.R., Morris, J.K., Wald, N.J. (1997) 'Environmental tobacco smoke and ischaemic heart disease: an evaluation of the evidence', *BMJ*, 315: 973–80.

Law, M.R., Thompson, S.G., Wald, N.J. (1994a) 'Assessing possible hazards of reducing serum cholesterol', *BMJ*, 308:373–9.

Law, M.R., Wu, T., Wald, N.J., Hackshaw, A., Thompson, S.G., Bailey, A. (1994b) 'Authors' reply', *BMJ*, 308: 1041.

Lawson, M. (1996) 'Icebergs and rocks and the "good" lie', *Guardian*, 24 June.

Layzell, S., Graffy, J (1998) *Evaluation of FWA's WellFamily Project*, London: Statham Grove Surgery.

Lea, R. (2000) *Healthcare in the UK: The Need for Reform*, London: Institute of Directors.

LeFanu, J. (1987) *Eat Your Heart Out*, London: Macmillan.

——(1994) 'A healthy diet – fact or fiction?' in *Health, Lifestyle and Environment*, London/New York: Social Affairs Unit/Manahattan Institute.

——(ed.) (1994) *Preventionitis*, London: Social Affairs Unit.

——(1994) *Environmental Alarums*, London: Social Affairs Unit.

——(1999) *The Rise and Fall of Modern Medicine*, London: Little, Brown.

Levitt, N. (1999) *Prometheus Bedevilled*, New Brunswick/New Jersey/London: Rutgers University Press.

Limerick (1998) *The Limerick Report*, The final report of the expert group to investigate cot death theories, London: DOH.

Lock, S. (1997) 'Medicine in the Second Half of the Twentieth Century', in I. Loudon (ed.) *Western Medicine*, Oxford: Oxford University Press.

Loudon, I. (ed.) (1997) *Western Medicine*, Oxford: Oxford University Press.

Lowry, S. (1993) *Medical Education*, London: BMJ.

Lupton, D. (1995) *The Imperative of Health*, London: Sage.

McCormick, J. (1996) 'Death of the personal doctor', *Lancet*, 348: 667–68 (7 September).

MacKeith, N. (1976) *Women's Health Handbook*, London: Expression.

MacKenzie, M.D. (1946) 'The World Health Organisation', *BMJ*, 21 September: 428–30.

McKeown, T. (1976a) *The Modern Rise of Population*, London: Edward Arnold.

——(1976b) *The Role of Medicine* (first edition), Oxford: Nuffield Hospitals Trust.

——(1979) *The Role of Medicine* (second edition), Oxford: Blackwell.

Marmot, M. (1994) 'The cholesterol papers', *BMJ*, 308: 351–2.

Marmot, M., Brunner, E. (1991) 'Alcohol and cardio-vascular disease: the status of the U-shaped curve', *BMJ*, 303: 565–8.

Marsch, L.A. (1998) 'The efficacy of methadone maintenance interventions in reducing illicit opiate use, HIV risk behaviour and criminality: a meta-analysis', *Addiction*, 93 (4): 515–32.

May, M., Brunsdon, E. (1994) 'Workplace care in the mixed economy of welfare', *Social Policy Review*, 6, London: Social Policy Association.

Maxwell, R. (1991) 'Preface' in A. Smith *et al.* (eds) *The Nation's Health*, London: King Edward's Hospital Fund for London.

Meadow, R. (1999) 'Unnatural sudden infant death', *Archives of Diseases of Childhood*, 80: 7–14.

Mechanic, D. (1997) 'The social context of health and disease and choices among health interests', in A.M. Brandt and P. Rozin (eds), *Morality and Health*, London: Routledge.

Medawar, P. (1986) *The Limits of Science*, Oxford: Oxford University Press.

Medical Council on Alcoholism (1987) *Hazardous Drinking: A Handbook for General Practitioners*, London: MCA.

Merrison (1975) *Report of the Committee of Inquiry into the Regulation of the Medical Profession* (Merrison Report), Cmnd 6018, London: HMSO.

Moon, G., Gillespie, R. (1995) *Society and Health*, London: Routledge.

Mooney, J. (1993) *The Hidden Figure: Domestic Violence in North London*, London: Middlesex University/Islington Council.

Mullan, P. (1999) *The Imaginary Time-Bomb*, London: IB Tauris.

Murphy, T. (1996) *Rethinking the War on Drugs*, Cork: Cork University Press.

Navarro, V. (1976) *Medicine Under Capitalism*, New York: Prodist.

Nettleton, S. (1995) *The Sociology of Health and Illness*, Cambridge: Polity.

Nicholl, J. (1992) 'Exercise, fitness and health', *BMJ*: 305: 645.

Nilsson, R. (1997) 'Is environmental tobacco smoke a risk factor for carcinoma of the lung?' in R. Bate (ed.) *What Risk*, London: Butter-worth/Heinemann.

Nolan, J.L. (1998) *The Therapeutic State*, New York: New York University Press.

North, R., Gorman, T. (1990) *Chickengate*, London: Institute of Economic Affairs Health and Welfare Unit.

Nottingham, J. (1999) 'Women must be given fully informed information about cervical screening', *BMJ*, 318: 1555–6.

Nuffield Institute for Health, Welsh Institute for Health and Social Care, London School of Hygiene and Tropical Medicine (1998) *The Health of the Nation – A Policy Assessed*, London: Stationery Office.

Oakley, A. (1976) 'Wisewoman and Medicine Man: Changes in the Management of Childbirth' in A. Oakley and J. Mitchell (eds) *The Rights and Wrongs of Women*, Harmondsworth: Penguin.

Omran, A. (1971) 'The Epidemiological Transition: A Theory of the Epidemiology of Population Change', *Millbank Memorial Fund Quarterly*, 49: 509–38.

OPCS (1990) *Mortality Statistics 1990*, London: HMSO.

Owen, D. (1976) 'Patient help thyself', *Sunday Times*, 3 October.

Peele, S. (1985) *The Meaning of Addiction*, San Francisco: Jossey Bass.

——(1995) *The Diseasing of America*, San Francisco: Jossey Bass.

Peterson, A., Lupton, D., (1996) *The New Public Health*, London: Sage.

Porter, D. (1999) *Health, Civilisation and the State*, London: Routledge.

Porter, R. (1997) *The Greatest Benefit to Mankind*, London: HarperCollins.

Power, M. (1994) *The Audit Explosion*, London: Demos.

——(1997) *The Audit Society: Rituals of Verification*, Oxford: Oxford University Press.

President of the Council (1995) *Tackling Drugs Together*, London: HMSO.

——(1998) *Tackling Drugs to Build a Better Britain*, London: HMSO.

Pringle, M., Laverty, J. (1993) 'A counsellor in every practice?', *BMJ*, 306: 2–3.

Public Health Alliance (1992) *The Health of the Nation: Challenges for a New Government*, Birmingham: PHA.

Public Health Laboratory Service (2000) *Aids/HIV Quarterly Surveillance Tables*, 45 (99) 4 (March), London: PHLS.

Quinn, M., Babb, P., Jones, J., Allen, E. (1999) 'Effect of screening on incidence of and mortality from cancer of the cervix in England: evaluation based on routinely collected statistics', *BMJ*, 318: 904–8.

Quinn, M., Babb, P.J., Jones, J. (1999) 'Authors' reply', *BMJ*, 319: 642.

Raffle, A.E. (1997) 'Informed participation in screening is essential', *BMJ*, 314: 1762–3.

Raffle, A.E., Alden, B., Mackenzie, E.D.F. (1995) 'Detection rates for abnormal cervical smears: what are we screening for?', *Lancet*, 345: 1469–73.

Ramsay, L.E., Yeo, W.W., Jackson, P.R. (1994) 'Effective diets are unpalatable', *BMJ*, 308: 1039.

Ratey, J., Johnson, C. (1997) *Shadow Syndromes*, London: Bantam.

Rees, J. (1996) 'The melanoma epidemic: artefact and reality', *BMJ*, 312: 137–8.

Rivett, G. (1998) *From Cradle to Grave*, London: Kings Fund.

Robbins, C. (ed.) (1987) *Health Promotion in North America*, London: Health Education Council/King Edward's Hospital Fund for London.

Rogers, L. (1995) 'Pioneer resigns over "useless" breast cancer tests', *Sunday Times*, 3 September.

Rose, G. (1985) 'Sick individuals and sick populations', *International Journal of Epidemiology*, 14: 32–38.

Rose, G., Marmot, M. (1981) 'Social class and coronary heart disease', *BMJ*, 45: 13–19.

Rosen, G. (1993) *A History of Public Health*, Baltimore: Johns Hopkins.

Rosenberg, C. (1997) 'Banishing risk: continuity and change in the moral managment of disease', in A.M. Brandt and P. Rozin (eds) *Morality and Health*, London: Routledge.

Royal College of General Practitioners (1988) *Alcohol – a Balanced View*, London: RCGP.

——(1996) *The Nature of General Medical Practice*, London: RCGP.

——(October 1999) *Good Medical Practice for General Practitioners*, London: RCGP.

——November 1999) *Revalidation for General Practice*, London: RCGP.

Royal College of Midwives (1997) *Domestic Abuse in Pregnancy. Position Paper 19*. London: Royal College of Midwives.

Royal College of Physicians (1962) *Smoking and Health*, London: Royal College of Physicians.

——(1971) *Smoking and Health Now*, London: Royal College of Physicians.

——(1987) *The Medical Consequence of Alcohol Abuse*, London: Tavistock.

——(1991) *Medical Aspects of Exercise, Benefits and Risks*, London: RCP.

——(2000) *Nicotine Addiction in Britain*, London: RCP.

Royal College of Physicians, Royal College of Psychiatrists, Royal College of General Practitioners (1995) *Alcohol and the Heart in Perspective*, London: RCP, RCPsych, RCGP.

Royal College of Psychiatrists (1986) *Our Favourite Drug: New Report on Alcohol and Alcohol-Related Problems*, London: Tavistock.

Sackett, D.L., Holland, W.W. (1975) 'Controversy in the detection of disease', *Lancet*, ii: 357–9.

Scott, B. (1997) 'Treatment expectations for drug users', *Substance Misuse Management in General Practice Newsletter*, 7: 1–3 (September).

Scott-Samuel, A. (1989) 'Building the new public health' in C.J. Martin and D.V. McQueen (eds) *Readings for a New Public Health*, Edinburgh: Edinburgh University Press.

Seddon, T. (2000) 'Explaining the drug-crime link: theoretical, policy and research issues', *Journal of Social Policy*, 29, 1, 95–107.

Sedgwick, P. (1982) *Psychopolitics*, London: Pluto.

Shaw, M., Dorling, D., Gordon, D., Davey Smith, G. (1999) *The Widening Gap*, Bristol: Policy Press.

Shilling, C. (1993) *The Body and Social Theory*, London: Sage.

Shorter, E. (1985) *Doctors and their Patients: A Social History*, New Brunswick/London: Transaction.

Shuster, S. (1992) 'Apocalypse now?' *BMJ*, 305: 200–1.

Sigerist, H. (1941) *Medicine and Human Welfare*, New Haven: Yale University Press.

Silagy, C., Mant, D., Fowler, G., Lancaster, T. (1999) 'Nicotine replacement therapy for smoking cessation', in *Cochrane Library*, Oxford: Update Software 1998, Issue 2.

Skrabanek, P. (1994) *The Death of Humane Medicine and the Rise of Coercive Healthism*, London: Social Affairs Unit.

Skrabanek, P., McCormick, J. (1989) *Follies and Fallacies in Medicine*, Tarragon Press.

Smeeth, L., Fowler, G. (1998) 'Nicotine replacement therapy for a healthier nation', *BMJ*, 317: 1266–7.

Smith, A., Jacobson, B., Whitehead, M. (eds) (1988) *The Nation's Health: A Strategy for the 1990s*; A Report from an Independent Inter-departmental Committee chaired by Professor Alwyn Smith, London: King Edward's Hospital Fund for London.

Smith, R. (1999) 'Managing the clinical performance of doctors', *BMJ*, 319: 1314–5.

Social Affairs Unit/Manhattan Institute (1991) *Health, Lifestyle and the Environment*, London/New York: SAU/Manhattan Institute.

Sontag, S. (1989) *Aids and its Metaphors*: London: Penguin.

Southall, D.P., Samuels, M.P. (1992) 'Reducing risks in the sudden infant death syndrome', *BMJ*, 304: 265–6.

Southgate, L., Pringle, M. (1999) 'Revalidation in the United Kingdom: general principles based on experience in general practice', *BMJ*, 319: 1180–3.

Starr, P. (1982) *The Social Transformation of American Medicine*, New York: Basic Books.

Steadman Rice, J. (1998) *A Disease of One's Own*, New Jersey: Transaction.

Stevenson, H.M., Burke, M. (1991) 'Bureaucratic logic in new social movement clothing', *Health Promotion International*, 6; 4: 281–90.

Steward, F., Wibberley, G. (1980) 'Drug innovation: what's slowing it down?', *Nature*, 284: 118–20.

Stimson, G.V., Hickman, M., Turnbull, P.J. (1998) 'Statistics on misuse of drugs have been misused', *BMJ*, 317: 1388.

Swales, J.D. (1995) 'The population paradox', *Journal of the Royal Society of Medicine*, 88: 605–6.

Syme, S.L., Alcalay, R. (1982) 'Control of cigarette smoking from a social perspective', *Annual Review of Public Health*, 3: 179–99.

Szasz, T. (1974 [1961]) *The Myth of Mental Illness* (revised edition), New York: Harper and Row.

Taylor, B., Miller, E., Farrington, C.P., Petropoulos, M.C., Favot-Mayaud, I., Li, J., Waight, P.A. (1999) 'Autism and measles, mumps and rubella vaccine: no epidemiological evidence for a causal association', *Lancet*, 353: (12 June).

Thomas, K. (1997) 'Health and morality in early modern England', in A.M. Brandt and P. Rozin (eds) *Morality and Health*, London: Routledge.

Thomas, L. (1979) *The Medusa and the Snail*, London: Penguin.

Thoreau, H.D. (1986) *Walden* and *Civil Disobedience* (first published separately in 1854 and 1849), London: Penguin Classics.

Timmins, N. (1995) *The Five Giants*, London: HarperCollins.

Toon, P. (1994) *What Is Good General Practice?*, Occasional Paper 65, London: RCGP.

——(1999) *Towards a Philosophy of General Practice*, Occasional Paper 78, London: RCGP.

Townsend, P., Davidson, N. (1988) *Inequalities in Health* (incorporating P. Townsend and N.Davidson (eds) *The Black Report* and Whitehead, M., *The Health Divide*), London: Pelican.

US Department of Health, Education and Welfare (1979) *Healthy People*, Washington, DC: US Government Printing Office.

——(1980) *Promoting Health, Preventing Disease*, Washington, DC: US Government Printing Office.

US Environmental Protection Agency (1992) *Respiratory Health Effects of Passive Smoking*, Washington, DC: EPA.

US Surgeon-General (1986) *The Health Consequences of Involuntary Smoking*, Rockville, MD: US Department of Health and Human Services.

——(1988) *The Health Consequences of Smoking, Nicotine Addiction*, Washington, DC: US Department of Health and Human Services.

Vaidya, J.S., Baum, M. (1999) 'Screening and mortality from cervical cancer', *BMJ*, 319: 642.

Vine, D.L., Hastings, G.E. (1994) 'Absolute risk more informative than relative risk', *BMJ*: 308: 1040.

Wainwright, D. (1996) 'The political transformation of the health inequalities debate', *Critical Social Policy 49*, 16 (4) 6–82.

Waitzkin, H. (1978) 'A Marxist view of medical care', *Annals of Internal Medicine*, 89: 264–78.

Wakefield, A.J., Murch, S.H., Anthony, A., Linnell, J., Casson, D.M., Malik, M., Berelowitz, M., Dhillon, A.P., Thomson, M.A., Harvey, P., Valentine, A., Davies, S.E., Walker-Smith, J.A. (1998) 'Ileal-lymphoid-nodular hyperplasia, non-specific colitis, and pervasive developmental disorder in children', *Lancet*, 351: 637–41.

Weatherall, D. (1995) *Science and the Quiet Art*, Oxford: Oxford University Press.

Webster, C. (1988) *The Health Services Since the War*, London: HMSO.

Wells, J. (1998) 'Mammography and the politics of randomised controlled trials', *BMJ*, 317: 1224–30.

Wessely, S., Hotopf, M., Sharpe, M. (1998) *Chronic Fatique and its Syndromes*, Oxford: Oxford University Press.

Whelan, P. (1997) 'Are we promoting stress and anxiety?', *BMJ*, 315: 1549–50.

White, I.R., McKie, M. (1997) 'Festive cheer for all?', *BMJ*, 315: 1638–9.

Wildavsky, A. (1977) 'Doing Better and Feeling Worse: The Political Pathology of Health Policy', *Daedalus*, 106 (Winter 1977).

——(1995) *But Is It True?*, Cambridge, Mass.: Harvard.

Wilkinson, R. (1996) *Unhealthy Societies*, London: Routledge.

Willis, J. (1995) *The Paradox of Progress*, London: Radcliffe.

Wilson, J.M.G., Jungner, G. (1968) *Principles and Practice of Screening for Disease*, Geneva: World Health Organisation.

Winnicott, D.W. (1965) *The family and individual development*, London: Tavistock.

Zola, I. (1972) 'Medicine as an institution of social control', *The Sociological Review*, November: 487–504.

INDEX